FASTING

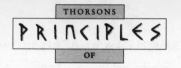

FASTING

LEON CHAITOW

Thorsons
An Imprint of HarperCollins*Publishers*

The publishers would like to thank
Jillie Collings for her suggestion for
the title of this series, *Principles of...*

Thorsons
An Imprint of HarperCollins*Publishers*
77–85 Fulham Palace Road
Hammersmith, London W6 8JB

1160 Battery Street
San Francisco, California 94111–1213

Published by Thorsons 1996
5 7 9 10 8 6 4 2

A catalogue record for this book
is available from the British Library

ISBN 0 7225 3306 3

Printed and bound in Great Britain by
Caledonian International Book Manufacturing Ltd, Glasgow

CONTENTS

CAUTION

The evidence offered in this book about the possible value of therapeutic fasting should be understood to be provided for information only, and not as a recommendation in any particular case for the use of fasting as a therapeutic intervention.

If any fast is undertaken for longer than 48 hours it is strongly suggested that a suitably qualified, competent and experienced health care professional (see Resources section) should be consulted for advice and to ensure that supervision is available.

Fasting is to be actively discouraged outside of a residential setting for anyone with an eating disorder (such as anorexia and bulimia) or who suffers from any form of mental disease which requires medication to control it. Fasting is particularly contraindicated for anyone who does not fully understand and agree with its application.

The author and publishers specifically caution against lengthy fasting (anything longer than two days) without expert supervision.

WHAT IS FASTING?

At the age of 12 I experienced acute abdominal pain, and a doctor advised immediate hospitalization for removal of my appendix. My mother had also asked for advice from my father's brother, a noted naturopath and chiropractor, Boris Chaitow (cousin of Stanley Lief, of whom more later).

My uncle Boris took the extraordinary – many would say irresponsibly foolhardy – step of advising against surgery, and placed me on a water fast. During the following 10 days I (a most unco-operative patient!) was subjected to the indignity of regular tepid enemas, as well as hot and cold packs and a water-only regime.

A few key facts are clearly embedded in my memory – that after the first day I lost all interest in and desire for food; that I detest enemas, and that I felt extremely well during the last week of the fast, with no sign of the agonizing pain previously experienced.

I am well aware that the whole enterprise could have turned out disastrously had my appendix ruptured, as the doctor had envisaged if surgery was delayed. But it did not, and I still have both it and a firm conviction based on personal experience of the value of therapeutic fasting. Incidentally, at the time of writing, Boris Chaitow is alive and well and just short of his 90th birthday.

Having subsequently trained in osteopathy and naturopathy (of which fasting forms an important element) I have over the years advised many patients with a variety of health complaints to fast – but have never had the nerve to risk what Boris (and my parents) risked with my appendicitis – nor do I recommend anyone else to do so.

FASTING DEFINED

Fasting is the avoidance – totally or partially – of the eating of food and liquid, except for pure water, for a particular period of time.

There are also a number of modified versions of fasting which allow the taking of juices, and even some foods, as part of their protocols. There are 'mono-diets' (single food fasting such as the 'grape cure'), dry fasts (eating dry rusks with minimal liquid intake, as in the 'Schroth Cure'), juice fasts and herb tea fasts.

In absolute terms, these methods are not really 'fasts' at all, but 'restricted diets'. However, since they offer some of the benefits of fasting (especially if repeated regularly) they are included as possible alternatives.

FASTING IS NOT STARVATION

Not eating does not mean that you are starving. There is, in most people, enough reserve food stored to last for many days – usually many weeks. So, during a controlled therapeutic fast the body does not use any of its essential tissues as fuel, but instead 'burns' or metabolizes fat stores. At the same time a variety of important detoxification and repair processes begin which are of immense value to health, and these are explained in detail in later chapters.

The use above of the word *controlled* is meant to indicate that there are 'right' and 'wrong' ways of fasting, and just what should and should not be done when a fast is undertaken (to ensure both safety and effectiveness) is very carefully outlined as we look at the long history and use of fasting for health.

Probably the most undesirable way to fast is if you have a particular health problem and stop eating, fail to drink sufficient water and/or continue to take non-essential medication. Note that insulin, thyroid hormone and, in some instances, prednisone are regarded as 'essential' if you have become dependent upon their continued use to the extent that stopping their intake could produce a violent and possibly fatal result.

The way a fast is conducted, and the way it is broken, are very important indeed, and you are urged to read all of this book, not just parts of it, and to fully appreciate the guidance offered before experimenting with a fast. Serious problems have been known to occur when rules are broken during fasts.

To effectively and safely use fasting as a means of restoring (and maintaining) good health, it is necessary to fully understand the self-healing functions of the body and how they operate. These are explained in this book, and once you have grasped them and are fully aware of the rules, the potential of this marvellous method of regeneration is open to you, should you choose to use it.

FIRST CHOICE IN FEVER

There is probably no more powerful healing method than therapeutic fasting when it is applied correctly and used responsibly and safely, since fasting does not impose a solution on the disturbed workings of the body, but allows it space and time, a

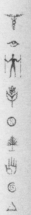

4   period of 'physiological rest', during which healing can occur naturally.

In acute conditions, most notably fevers and infections, it should be the first choice of health care, since fasting dramatically increases the efficiency of the immune function, at least for the first 24 to 36 hours.

In chronic conditions, such as heart disease, rheumatoid arthritis, ulcerative colitis, psoriasis and eczema, there is a huge amount of evidence showing that controlled and supervised fasting can help such stubborn and sometimes life-threatening conditions to clear completely.

LONG OR SHORT FASTS?

In the UK, between the First and Second World Wars, Stanley Lief ND, DC, the gifted naturopathic healer, supervised thousands of successful lengthy fasts at Champneys, the health resort in Hertfordshire which he ran for over 30 years. The longest fast recorded at Champneys lasted for over three months (95 days), the outcome of which was the patient's complete recovery from chronic ill-health (I know because I met the 'patient' some 30 years later during my own working period at Champneys in the early 1960s).

In the USA, Herbert Shelton, the pioneer practitioner of Natural Hygiene, also initiated and supervised numerous fasts in severely ill patients, often with amazing results.

If these two practitioners, and their countless followers, achieved such wonderful results, why are we not told more of fasting as a means of healing?

Well, to be sure, we are, but you have to search for reports of fasting benefits in the medical journals, where only now and then evidence appears which supports the results claimed for this most ancient, efficient and potentially inexpensive of healing methods.

In 1991, for example, the prestigious medical journal *The Lancet* published the results of a one-year study of patients with rheumatoid arthritis who had been treated by means of fasting and a vegetarian diet.

WHAT PREVENTS THE WIDER USE OF FASTING?

The results of fasting patients with rheumatoid arthritis were so good that there can now be no doubt at all that fasting should be the treatment of choice for this condition – and for almost all auto-immune conditions in which the body's defence systems attack parts of itself. That few rheumatologists employ fasting for their patients is indicative of both the lack of awareness of such studies by most doctors, and the power of the pervading idea that we have to 'take something' to assuage symptoms, or to control pain and disability.

To be fair, even when faced with the evidence of the value of fasting, many people will still opt for the dubious convenience of swallowing pills and potions rather than doing something for themselves to restore their health by methods which are slow, sometimes uncomfortable, and which involve effort and will-power.

Fasting involves commitment, acceptance of responsibility for getting well, and a dedicated sense of purpose, and these qualities are not always the first to present themselves when we are faced with a choice between a means of treatment which someone may not fully understand and something which has the backing of current medical authority.

This is why it is so important to be fully aware of the facts about fasting – including its drawbacks, requirements, benefits and potentials before embarking on its use.

DRAWBACKS

There are several potential drawbacks to fasting which need to be highlighted at the outset.

- Long fasts (of more than two days) require supervision by a suitably qualified health care professional. This raises the question of cost and time, since staying in a clinic (often for many weeks) where appropriate supervision is available, or paying for regular home visits over an extended period of time, could prove very expensive. Also, since awareness of the value of fasting is limited amongst orthodox medical practitioners, a level of determination is sometimes required to find someone suitably qualified. You will need to look for a fully trained naturopath, a German 'heilpraktiker', an Ayurvedic (traditional Indian medicine) practitioner or a clinical ecologist.

- Many people find the whole idea of stopping eating for weeks on end too bizarre to contemplate, and they would undoubtedly have anxieties which could make the starting of such a process unwise. For the best results it is essential that the person fasting should be comfortable with the idea, aware of the processes involved, and happy to participate in the healing process.

- There is evidence to suggest that because of the increase in levels of environmental toxicity, to which we are all exposed in one way or another, the progress of a fast is far less predictable than it was just 50 years ago when Lief and Shelton were at the peak of their practice of therapeutic fasting.

During a fast, such pollutants and residues from previous medical treatment (e.g. steroid medication) or from 'social' use (e.g. tobacco and other drugs) can be released when fat stores are used up – fat is where many toxins are safely stored or 'dumped' by a body overloaded with toxic debris – possibly producing reactions of an unpredictable nature as a 'cocktail' of chemicals hits the bloodstream.

AN EFFECTIVE COMPROMISE

Given the above drawbacks, which may preclude many from enjoying the benefits of fasting, what modifications are possible which might allow for fasting to be inexpensively and safely applied?

To avoid expense, to make the process less intimidating and, above all, to ensure greater safety – regular short fasts are suggested as an alternative to lengthy or 'open-ended' fasts.

The process of detoxification and healing is bound to be less dramatic with this alternative, but it is really the only option open if you cannot afford the expense or the time (leaving out the toxic danger referred to) needed for an open-ended, supervised fast.

WHAT YOU NEED TO KNOW

In this compact but complete introduction to fasting for both health enhancement and spiritual growth, the different techniques and modifications of fasting (long and short) are explained, backed up by research evidence for its use in the treatment of various ailments. It also includes the pros and cons of using fasting as part of a weight maintenance strategy.

Associated detoxification methods are outlined – including various forms of hydrotherapy and the vexed question of supplementation (should you or shouldn't you during a fast?).

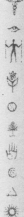

Indications and contraindications to fasting are spelled out, so that by the end you will know when fasting should be used, when it is inappropriate, how to plan, prepare for and start a fast.

You will also have a good idea of what benefits, signs and symptoms to expect on a fast, what to do about breaking the fast (a very important consideration) as well as how often and for how long to fast, taking into account your age, health status, weight, etc.

Evidence is also presented to explain an unexpected bonus from fasting – the increased production of growth hormone (HGH) by the pituitary gland, which helps to retard the ageing process.

For most people, fasting can be a revitalizing experience, restoring energy and a clear mind, as well as helping to remove a host of minor symptoms, while encouraging the self-healing mechanisms of the body to regenerate and rebuild a level of well-being you have probably all but forgotten.

FASTING – ANCIENT
AND MODERN

Partial or total fasting has been used for thousands of years by many religions and cultures as a means of increasing spiritual awareness and religious observation. For example, in Islamic tradition the period of Ramadan is characterized by complete abstinence from food or water during daylight hours for a period of a month. In the Jewish religion a fast day (no food or water) occurs during the 'Day of Atonement' (Yom Kippur) and yeasted grain products are avoided during the feast of the Passover, while Christianity has its Lent period when consumption of animal products are restricted prior to Easter.

Biblical descriptions of lengthy fasts are common, with the emphasis on the heightened levels of spiritual awareness that they lead to, and texts also exist showing fasting to be part of pagan ritual, for instance in classical Greek tradition hundreds of years before the Christian era.[1]

FASTING FOR HEALTH [2, 3]

Fasting as a health enhancing method also dates back to prehistory, with records of the great physician Hippocrates employing fasts as part of his healing regime for many patients.

'When one feeds a sick person, one only feeds the sickness.'
(*Hippocrates 460–377 BC*)

In more recent times the use of fasting as a therapeutic measure has been most widespread in Germany, the UK, Scandinavia and the USA. In these countries in particular there has been a good deal of research which shows the value of fasting in a wide range of diseases, some of which is recounted below.

One of the first doctors to widely advocate fasting in the USA was Isaac Jennings (1788–1874) who eventually abandoned the use of drugs and relied on a programme of vegetarian eating, pure water, sunshine, exercise, emotional balance, rest and fasting to bring about a restoration of health in his patients. With the assistance of a Presbyterian preacher, Sylvester Graham, Jennings promoted his Natural Hygienic methods which became extremely popular as an alternative to the indiscriminate and dangerous drugs in use at the time (early 1820s).

At much the same time in Germany and other parts of Europe the development of a Nature Cure tradition of healing closely mirrored that of the Hygienists, with priests such as Father Kneipp promoting both herbal methods, hydrotherapy and fasting. Towards the end of the nineteenth century the German physicians Henry Lindlahr and Benjamin Lust took these methods to the USA where, with aspects of the Hygienist concept, they and other doctors using the German tradition developed what became Naturopathic Medicine, which had fasting as one of its core strategies (along with dietary reform, herbal medicine, hydrotherapy, physical exercise and manual methods) of health promotion.

Dr John Kellogg (of corn-flake fame), with his vast Battle Creek Sanatorium (where there were over a thousand patients resident at any one time – most of them fasting), and John Tilden MD were two of the leading American doctors to promote fasting during the first half of this century in the USA.

Tilden's philosophy was summarized in his book *Toxaemia – the basic cause of disease*, in which he wrote:

> Every disease is built within the mind and body by enervating habits. A fast, rest in bed and giving up the enervating habits, mental and physical, will allow nature to eliminate the accumulated toxins, then, if enervating habits are given up, and rational living habits adopted, health will come to stay.

Tilden was emphasizing the main philosophical core of natural healing, that the body is self-healing if it is given the chance, and that the chance comes most effectively when the causes of the illness are removed ('giving up enervating habits') and the body is given the chance to recover ('fast and rest').

The naturopathic tradition in the USA is now well established, with three seats of higher education issuing doctorates in the subject (Naturopathic schools in Portland, Oregon; Seattle, Washington; and Scottsdale, Arizona). Graduates of these are recognized in approximately a quarter of the states of the USA as primary care physicians. The Bastyr College in Seattle, which became Bastyr University in 1994, is arguably the most dynamic of these training establishments, and is named after the last of the great American pioneers of naturopathy, John Bastyr, who died in 1995 at the age of 83.[4]

It was Stanley Lief, ND, DC, who brought naturopathic concepts and methods to the UK just before the First World War. His enthusiastic, widespread and highly successful application of 'the fasting cure' at Champneys Health Resort between 1925 and the late 1950s, helped to promote natural healing in Britain. Lief and his cousin Boris Chaitow, ND, DC, and subsequently Lief's son Peter, established modern naturopathic awareness in Britain. The long-term professional training of naturopaths in Britain was guaranteed thanks to Lief's founding of the British College of

Naturopathy and Osteopathy in London, where a full-time four-year degree course in osteopathy (validated by the University of Westminster) also contains a sound naturopathic education which incorporates training in the use of therapeutic fasting.

CLINICAL RESEARCH

Fasting research was first begun in the late nineteenth century, with 40-day fasts being closely monitored and the physiological and metabolic effects which took place being carefully recorded. For example, a report in the *British Medical Journal* in 1880[5] outlines the effects of a 40-day water fast on a Dr Tanner.

In the early twentieth century, therapeutic fasting – where patients were treated using the method – began to be reported in medical journals and in 1910 a report by Dr Guelpa appeared in the *British Medical Journal*[6] on the benefits of fasting in diabetes (see below).

WHEN DOES FASTING STOP AND STARVATION START?

The difference between fasting and starvation was the subject of much early research, and it has continued to exercise minds in subsequent concerted and lengthy studies. The conclusions drawn are that, in instances of food deprivation, starvation cannot be said to begin until all the body's fat stores have been used up, and significant protein breakdown has occurred.

Research shows that an average individual weighing 154 lb (11 stone/70 kg) has fat stores adequate for maintaining calorie requirements for between two and three months (calorie usage will vary with the basic metabolic rate of the individual and the amount of activity undertaken during a fast). When fat stores are used up there remains a store of protein which, as a rule, can maintain calorie levels for a few weeks longer before essential proteins from the vital organs start to be used. There are many signs which indicate when this threshold has been passed, when fasting which is beneficial has ended and when starvation which can kill has started.[7, 8]

WHAT DISEASES ARE HELPED BY FASTING?

The benefits of fasting in the treatment of **diabetes** were first revealed in research conducted by Dr G. Guelpa in 1910[6], and in 1915 Dr F. Allen showed that fasting could normalize the blood sugar levels of a diabetic, as well as improve associated gangrene.[9] Since then studies into this particular therapeutic potential of fasting have continued.[10]

Various medical papers have been published describing clinical trials showing how patients with **epilepsy** can be helped by fasting. Controlled fasting was found to reduce the length, severity and number of seizures.[11]

The use of fasting in **obesity** has not unnaturally received a great deal of attention. In one famous case, reported in 1973[12], a man fasted for over a year and lost 276 lb (19.7 stone/125 kg). Despite the success of this particular case, and while there is always an obvious and sometimes dramatic weight loss in response to fasting – research shows that for every pound lost more than half is fat, just over a quarter is protein and the rest water and salt – this method alone is not recommended. There is general agreement that a fasting weight loss programme should include counselling and lifestyle modification if weight loss is to be maintained.

In one stringent study which lasted over seven years, involving over 120 obese patients who fasted for an average of two months, it was shown that after between two and three years half the patients had reverted to their previous weight, and after seven years and three months 90 per cent of the patients weighed what they did before the fast.[13]

A great deal of research has verified the value of fasting in the treatment of **heart disease** and **high blood pressure**. In the 1960s and 1970s a host of reports appeared in the medical press on how fasting had been shown to reduce the levels of undesirable fats in the bloodstream, to lower high blood pressure, to reduce cholesterol levels, to bring about improvements in cases of atheroma and to alleviate congestive heart failure.[14, 15]

The use of fasting as a treatment for acute **pancreatitis** was compared with the standard medical treatment for this condition (nasogastric suction and cimetidine) in a clinical study conducted in 1984 involving 88 patients. Results concluded that:

> Fasting alone should be used initially as the simpler and more economical therapy. Neither nasogastric suction nor cimetidine offer any advantage over fasting alone in the treatment of mild to moderate acute pancreatitis, of whatever cause.[16]

Chemical toxicity has been successfully treated using fasting – for example, when toxic cooking oil containing the rice oil contaminant PCB was consumed, patients were reported to have relief from their symptoms, sometimes dramatically so, after between seven and 10 days of fasting.[17]

A most important caution relevant to the above case needs to be reiterated here, since it is pointed out that when fat is mobilized during a fast, fat soluble toxins (such as DDT) can reach very high, and potentially lethal, levels in the bloodstream. This highlights the advice given in the first chapter of this book, which is that in today's world, and especially if toxic levels are high (previous exposure to chemicals, medical and other drugs, for example), repetitive short fasts are a safer way forward than lengthy fasts. If long fasts (anything over four days) are chosen then these must *always* be under clinical supervision, including monitoring for blood toxaemia.

Patients with those conditions known as **auto-immune diseases**, which include lupus, ankylosing spondylitis, rheumatoid arthritis, glomerulonephritis (kidney disease) amongst others, have shown marked benefits when fasting has been used in their treatment. In **glomerulonephritis**, for example, when fasting was used in the early stages the overall prognosis was improved. The researchers stated: 'all patients with acute glomerulonephritis should fast.'[18]

Treatment by fasting of another auto-immune disease, **rheumatoid arthritis**, was shown in a recent Scandinavian study to be very effective indeed. This study is worth looking at in a little more detail than those mentioned above, since it brings out a number of the possible benefits which fasting has to offer.

A one-year study was undertaken in which patients with well established rheumatoid arthritis were either treated using standard medical methods or a month of periodic fasting followed by a dairy free vegetarian diet. Many tests were performed to measure the changes in the blood status and symptom pictures of the two groups, and the examining doctors were unaware of which group the patient they were evaluating belonged to.

After the fast period, foods were reintroduced very carefully, with one 'new' food being started every second day and a watch being kept on any reaction to it (stiffness, swelling, etc.). If any symptom did appear, the food was left out for another week then tried again, and if a second reaction occurred (within 48 hours of the food being eaten) it was left out completely for the rest of the one-year study.

This part of the study suggests the possibility that in auto-immune disease there may be undesirable absorption through the intestinal wall of food particles which then provoke the immune system into an over-reaction, leading to some or all of the symptoms. Certainly, the fast would deny the chance of this happening since no food is being taken.

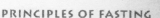

On restarting eating, the careful monitoring of foods for reactions allows for the accurate identification of culprit foods so that they can be eliminated from the diet altogether.

This process explains why those doctors specializing in allergy, often called Clinical Ecologists, use fasting as their main method of clearing the system of all allergen foods before starting the process of 'challenge' or testing, to see what provokes symptoms to return.

It is generally thought by Clinical Ecologists that five days is the length of time needed to completely clear the body of all traces of such foods, and the five-day fast is, therefore, a standard approach used by them.

That there are probably other benefits which derive from fasting, such as improved function of elimination and detoxification, is commonly ignored by this group of doctors. However, their unawareness or non-acceptance does not stop such additional fasting benefits from happening.

In the study involving the patients with rheumatoid arthritis, after one month of fasting and the gradual reintroduction of foods (but with no eggs, dairy foods, meat, fish, refined sugar, alcohol, tea and coffee for at least three months) remarkable benefits in the fasting/vegetarian group of patients were observed and reported. Joints were less stiff, swollen and painful and strength was increased, while blood tests showed lower sedimentation rates and reduction in markers which indicate rheumatoid activity. These benefits were still present after a year – in all the many signs and indications which were measured – when compared to those patients receiving standard medical attention.[19]

Were these benefits simply the result of the elimination of particular foods? Or is there overall a more efficient immune response after fasting? In an earlier study, which showed similar benefits of fasting in the treatment of auto-immune disease, D. R. Panush suggested that the answer to both questions is possibly yes:

Nutritional modification (fasting) might alter immune responsiveness and thereby effect manifestations of rheumatic diseases; or rheumatic disease may be a manifestation of food allergy or hypersensitivity.

Fasting might, in other words, improve the way the body works, or it might just remove from the scene the irritants to which the immune system is reacting...or both.[20]

Joel Fuhrman, MD, who strongly advocates fasting, has had success in treating a wide range of diseases, including auto-immune problems, using fasting. He reports that systemic lupus erythematosus (SLE) responds well to this approach.

As soon as a person is diagnosed with lupus, they should immediately begin a medically supervised fast to initiate remission. Breaking the fast carefully under proper guidance is extremely important. Upon completion of the fast the following foods should be avoided for a prolonged period of time: 1. All animal foods, including dairy products and eggs; 2. All legumes except peas and lima beans; 3. Celery, corn, alfalfa sprouts, mushrooms, spinach and figs.

The reason for avoiding these plant foods is that they contain a variety of chemicals which have been shown to cause reactions which can aggravate lupus and other auto-immune diseases.[21, 22, 23]

OTHER CONDITIONS AND FASTING

Many other diseases and problems have been successfully treated using fasting as the main therapeutic tool. These include **psoriasis**, the often intractable skin condition. Scandinavian research showed that benefits could be obtained by fasting (eight out of 10 patients improved markedly after a 7–10 day fast) and a vegetarian diet, but that the condition returned if the diet reverted to the previous pattern.[24]

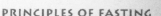

Auto-immune bowel diseases such as **ulcerative colitis** and **Crohn's disease** have responded extremely well to fasting and modified fasting (where liquid containing vitamins, minerals and some glucose was taken, but no food at all). In one study 84 per cent of those patients with Crohn's disease who were treated with fasting went into remission. Just as in the way rheumatoid arthritis was treated (see above), after the fast, foods (usually cooked for ease of digestion) were slowly reintroduced, and eliminated if there was any sign of diarrhoea or pain. Only 30 per cent of the patients with Crohn's disease who went into remission on the fast had relapses, whereas 66 per cent of those who were treated with cortisone type medication had relapses. The most provocative foods for irritable bowel diseases of this type are dairy products, most notably cow's milk, tea, coffee, chocolate, corn, wheat, rye, apples, oats and mushrooms.[25]

Among the many other conditions for which there is evidence of a useful role for fasting are **eczema**[26], **bronchial asthma**[27] and a variety of mental illness, including **schizophrenia**. Russia has been the country where mental illness has been most widely treated using fasting, most often by Professor Serge Nikoliav of the Moscow Psychiatric Institute. He has, with great success, treated over 6000 patients for chronic refractory schizophrenia by means of water fasts which run from 25 to 300 days (often accompanied by daily aerobic exercise).[28, 29]

Fasting for health is natural, efficient and, given the caveats already mentioned, safe. There are few conditions which cannot benefit from it and, as the brief survey in this chapter indicates, there is ample clinical evidence of its success.

The reason for this is that it allows healing to occur, and does not *impose* a solution on the body which, through its well-known homoeostatic (self-regulating) mechanisms, has an innate ability to normalize itself if it is given the chance. Fasting gives it that chance.

THE EFFECTS OF FASTING

Your mind–body is equipped to defend itself against, and cope with, invading micro-organisms, toxic materials, changes in temperature, unpleasant situations and a bewildering variety of stresses and strains of a mechanical, biochemical and emotional nature. For our entire lives we are in a state of adaptation, as the struggle to retain equilibrium continues.

Your body repairs itself given the chance – broken bones mend, cuts heal and the vast majority of infections are dealt with efficiently and without symptoms. Even when symptoms appear they are often only evidence of the body doing its self-repair and self-healing work. Fever, inflammation, diarrhoea, vomiting – are all evidence of the immune and other repair systems of the body performing their survival tasks.

Many emotions, such as anxiety and depression are only evidence of excessive degrees of perfectly normal emotions. It would be abnormal not to feel anxious in a situation of danger – however, an excessive amount of anxiety is not normal.

In just the same way, allergies are often evidence of an over-reaction on the part of the defence systems of the body to undesirable substances to which some reaction is perfectly normal.

Without fever, the body could not deal with invading microbes, viruses, parasites, etc. Without inflammatory processes, repair of damaged tissues could not take place. Without the ability to rapidly purge ourselves of the danger (vomiting, diarrhoea, etc.) poisons could rapidly kill us...and so on.

On a less dramatic scale we can see that a host of stress factors are making demands on our adaptation and repair processes all the time – both emotionally and biochemically – through the toxic exposure to which we are subject, the relative denatured quality of our food, the major emotional stresses of modern life – whether involving economics, family, relationships, employment or simply the hustle and rush of late twentieth century urban existence.

These multiple and complex adaptive demands can ultimately overwhelm our capacity for adaptation – especially if they are interacting on a mind–body complex which has inherited imbalances and weaknesses from the start.

A gradual decline in health therefore becomes an inevitable outcome, often signalled by the onset of what has been called 'vertical ill-health' in which we develop a range of minor symptoms which are not severe enough to send us to bed (horizontal ill-health) and which are seen as 'normal' because so many others have the same problems – ranging from digestive problems to skin complaints, headaches, disturbed sleep, aches and pains, etc.

WHAT'S TO BE DONE ABOUT THE STRESS OF LIFE?

There are only three strategies which can offer a beneficial change to the inevitable decline in health caused by biochemical, mechanical (posture, etc.) and emotional stressors impacting your defence systems:

1) You can try to remove the causes (eat better, exercise better, sleep better, relax more, etc.) and so reduce the demands being made on the adaptive, repair and defence capabilities of your body.

2) You can try to improve the adaptive, repair and defence capabilities of your body by methods which enhance immune and repair functions.

3) You can treat the symptoms – either in a way which causes no new problems (the ideal) or in ways which mask symptoms and actually create new problems. Examples of this are the use of anti-inflammatory drugs for arthritis, pain killers for a headache, antacid medication for indigestion – all of which can ease symptoms but do nothing to remove causes, and as a rule create side-effects and therefore new problems for the body to deal with.

In summary, we can try to reduce the stress load, and/or improve our ability to handle it, or we can try to palliate the effects of our handling of the load – well or badly – or, of course, we can choose to do nothing and simply crumble under the onslaught.

NATURAL HEALING OBJECTIVES

Unlike the use of medication and much surgical intervention which *imposes* solutions, or which makes forced alterations to the situation, natural healing methods start by respecting the self-healing (homoeostatic) potentials of the body.

This is sometimes referred to as *vis medicatrix naturae* or the 'healing power of nature'. In German texts it is often referred to as 'awakening the physician within', and in more scientific terminology as 'enhancing homoeostasis'.

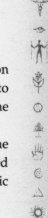

By whatever name, such methods appear to work by allowing space, giving a healing opportunity and doing the opposite of *forcing* a solution.

Fasting sits at the centre of such approaches, along with relaxation and meditation methods, the use of relaxing hydrotherapy methods such as the 'neutral bath' (see Chapter 6), the use of non-specific bodywork ('wellness massage' and aromatherapy relaxation methods, for example) and employment of techniques which have a balancing, harmonizing, normalizing influence – including some herbal and acupuncture methods.

None of these methods, in themselves, is 'curative', but all allow a healing potential to operate more efficiently because they offer the body–mind complex essential time, space and reduced demands, which encourages normalization and recovery, irrespective of whatever is wrong.

This is not to say that problems can be completely removed in all cases, since in many instances the processes that have already taken place will have created so much change, so much damage, that the best that can be hoped for is that matters do not get worse, or that there is a marginal improvement. This is, nevertheless, an infinitely better outcome than a steady decline into ever more ill health.

Trevor Salloum ND, a naturopathic practitioner, describes the benefits of fasting as:

…decreased weight, clearer skin, increased elimination, tissue repair, decreased pain and inflammation, increased concentration, relaxation, plus spare time and savings in the cost of food. Perhaps the greatest benefit is the satisfaction that you are taking a major role in improving your health.[1]

Apart from having to constantly adapt to the stress of life, another inevitable factor is always at work which makes demands on our adaptive processes – ageing.

There are a number of competing theories as to just what constitutes the mechanics of the ageing process, but there is increasing agreement that it is probably a combination of interacting elements – all happening at the same time. This was neatly summarized in *Newsweek* (5 March 1990) by journalists Sharon Begley and Mary Hager:

> One theory holds that the changes that accompany ageing are the inevitable result of life itself. DNA, the molecule of heredity, occasionally makes mistakes as it goes about its business of synthesizing proteins; metabolism produces toxic avengers (free radicals) that turn lipids [fats] in our cells rancid and proteins 'rusty'. This damage accumulates until the organism falls apart like an old jalopy...
>
> The other theory argues that ageing is genetic, programmed into the organism like puberty. There is evidence for both sides.

So we either gradually start to malfunction and fall apart because of wear and tear and the effects of accumulated toxic materials, and/or the whole process is as inevitable as growth, puberty and the menopause – it is preprogrammed in our cells.

Research into how to slow down this inevitable process has been focusing ever greater attention on to what has been termed 'calorie restriction' as a means of successfully reversing (or at least slowing) the decline into decrepitude and death.

The principle researchers in this field are Americans Richard Weindruch PhD and Roy Walford MD.[2] I have summarized their work and added other evidence to support the value of

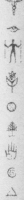

'calorie restriction' (which includes the use of fasting, mono-diets and exclusion/elimination diets) in my own book on the subject, *Natural Life Extension*.[3]

The evidence is overwhelming that dietary restriction is the only factor which consistently, and in all species increases the lifespan of experimental animals – ranging from mammals to fruit flies.

Such benefits are produced by a whole range of influences, it seems. Dietary restriction, including periodic fasting and living on a reduced calorie intake (while ensuring complete nutrient intake) as compared with the average diet, has a number of effects:

- There is a reduction in the core temperature of the body (such as occurs in a bear that is hibernating). The basic metabolic rate slows down which means that the rate at which the body functions and 'burns' energy slows down. This is a key requirement of any anti-ageing approach. A similar but more transient reduction in the core temperature of the body can also be achieved by deep meditation methods.

- There is a reduction in the build up of toxic wastes and therefore a lessening of free radical activity. Free radicals are the molecules which cause most tissue damage (arthritis, arterial disease, etc.). This is the same oxidation process that occurs when rubber perishes, fats become rancid, metals rust or an apple turns brown when exposed to the air.

This process can be reduced by either ensuring fewer free radical molecules are present in our tissues, which a restricted diet does, or by increasing the presence in our tissues of antioxidant nutrients (vitamins A, C and E, etc.) which the patterns of eating associated with fasting and detoxification also ensure.

- Production of protein for replacement of our damaged cells (protein synthesis is a constant process throughout life) occurs more efficiently when someone is on a restricted dietary pattern, including fasting, because fewer 'mistakes' are made by the DNA/RNA genetic controls which govern this process. If new protein is manufactured more efficiently tissues will be healthier, less prone to oxidation damage, more pliable and less likely to form what are scientifically called cross-linkages ('wrinkling' to you and I).

- Immune function and hormone production are seen to be more efficient during dietary restriction, and this includes that most important anti-ageing hormone, produced by the pituitary gland, human growth hormone (HGH) – production of which is also encouraged by exercise and sound sleep.

So, a pattern of eating and living which includes periodic fasting, mono-diets or detoxification periods, as described in this book (and ideally which also discourages a high calorie diet), is likely to enhance health as well as retard the ageing process via all the means described – slower metabolic rate, reduced free radical activity, better protein synthesis and enhanced immune function, combined with greater growth hormone levels.

These are not theories but facts, and the proof is there for you to test for yourself.

WHEN TO AND WHEN NOT TO FAST

Since fasting has no specific aim, but rather has a general potential to enhance the function of all the organs and systems, it could be seen as being universally applicable, and it is – almost.

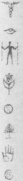

The following quotation, which is consistent with my own experience, is from the writing of Alex Burton ND, DO, who is one of the leading currently practicing proponents of fasting:

> I have found few health problems which are absolute contraindications to fasting. In my experience, if the need is evident, the only genuine contraindication is fear…As for the other conditions often mentioned [as contraindications], e.g. kidney disease, heart impairment, TB, etc., they merely require extreme caution, because of the limits imposed by pathology, but they are not inexorable contraindications.[4]

One of the priorities when trying to decide on a therapeutic approach needs to be that we do not make matters worse, and that new problems are not created.

Fasting for longer than two days can hardly ever cause harm, although some short-term symptoms might be noted. Some experts say that up to five days of unsupervised fasting is acceptable. However, I disagree and insist that no-one fasts for longer than four days without advice and supervision from a qualified health care professional, just in case there are unpredictable reactions.

WHAT ARE THE RISKS?

In the medical literature there are reports of thousands of clinical trials of fasting, usually involving severely ill patients often with life-threatening conditions, but only seven cases of death are recorded, and in five of these, drugs were administered during the fast – something which is quite definitely contraindicated.[4, 5, 6, 7, 8]

As Joel Fuhrman MD explains:

If we look at the details of these cases we can clearly see that the individuals were fasted improperly, using multiple drugs during the fast, in patients who had heart failure and kidney disease prior to the fast…[some of] these patients drank unrestricted amounts of coffee, tea and fruit juice during the fast and were given digoxin, diuretics and anticoagulants. These were not total fasts, and might more appropriately be called coffee and fruit juice feasts.

A statement taken from the ultra-cautious and medically conservative journal *The Lancet*[9] helps to put into context the relative danger:

Fasting short of emaciation is not hazardous. If death results, reasons other than those of the fast should be considered before concluding that all supervised fasts should be discouraged.

And remember that *none* of these tragedies was related to short-term fasting, which is the tactic highly recommended in this book for home use. It is worth repeating that *all* long-term fasting needs to be performed under supervision by a qualified and experienced health care professional.

CONTRAINDICATIONS TO FASTING BEYOND 48 HOURS

- **Emaciation**. Anyone who is severely underweight for any reason should not fast for long periods. However, controlled short fasts can assist in normalizing reasons for the emaciation in some cases (malabsorption problems, for example). If emaciation is because of advanced cancer, TB or AIDS or to an eating disorder such as anorexia, then fasting of any sort should not be undertaken.

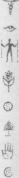

- **Fasting during pregnancy**. This could be dangerous for the foetus in some instances – especially if the woman is diabetic. Any fasting of a pregnant woman should be under strictly controlled and supervised conditions. Fasting is contraindicated when breast feeding, since milk flow is likely to cease and will be difficult to start again.

- **Fasting during menstruation**. It may be a good idea to avoid fasting just before or during menstruation as the detoxification process may result in an increased flow, increased discomfort or a delay in onset of the period.

- **Type l diabetics** should not be fasted according to many experts. However, some allow fasting as long as glucose levels are tested frequently and insulin intake adjusted according to lowered needs during a fast. **Type ll diabetics** should also be checked regularly, and they will probably find that sugar levels are normalized during the fast.

- **Infants** should not be fasted for longer than two days, and they seldom need even that length of time to respond well to this method of health promotion. There is seldom any reason for avoiding a short fast (36 to 48 hours) in a child of any age, should this be indicated (infection, digestive upset, skin reaction, etc.).

- **Kidney failure** is thought to be a sound reason for avoiding fasting since it makes excessive demands on the remaining kidney function. However, under controlled conditions short fasts can be helpful in such cases.

- **Medium-chain acyl CoA dehydrogenase** (MCAD) deficiency is a very rare enzyme defect which makes it difficult for the body to process the fatty acids which are mobilized during a fast. In such cases urine may appear light in colour which is unusual during a fast, when a great deal of waste (ketones) are being processed. Extreme lethargy and vomiting are early signs. Such problems would only present a danger on a long fast, and not during a short (48 hour) fast because the mobilization of fats would not be advanced until after some days of fasting.

- Long fasts are contraindicated in anyone with severe **liver disease** or severe **anaemia**. However, repetitive short fasts may be beneficial as part of an overall strategy to assist or normalize such problems.

- There are strong contraindications to even short-term fasting for anyone who is taking **prescription drugs**, as unpredictable reactions could occur. This is particularly true of anyone taking steroid medication, or who has taken steroid medication in the past for long periods. A similar caution is required regarding anyone taking forms of hormone replacement, such as in cases of underactive thyroid.

In all such cases (where steroid-hormone medication is current or has been prolonged) supervision of the fast in a controlled environment is essential, whether or not weaning from the medication has been possible prior to the fast.

Physician Joel Fuhrman, MD, explains his approach to patients on medication if he wishes to have them fast:

Normally, I taper medication as the patient adopts a healthy diet and postpone the fast until it is safe to discontinue most medication...If patients cannot reduce their dependency on such agents [toxic drugs which combined with fasting can cause toxic insult

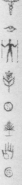

to the kidneys] through dietary and nutritional management prior to the fast, they are not suitable candidates for a fast.[10]

Among the forms of prescription medication which indicate that fasting should be avoided are the current use of antidepressants, non-steroidal-anti-inflammatory drugs, aspirin, oral hypoglycaemic drugs, anti-coagulant drugs, chemotherapeutic drugs and anti-hypertensive medication.

Once these have been safely stopped, with a physician's approval, fasting can begin. However, if the fast is to last for more than 48 hours, supervision is suggested.

- Anyone habitually using alcohol, tobacco, or other drugs should be very carefully detoxified (as well as stopping the habit) before any long-term fasting is considered. All signs of withdrawal should have abated before fasting is used, and careful monitoring should be continued throughout long-fasts. Short fasts, interspersed with other detoxification methods (see Chapter 5) are preferable.

- No-one who is afraid of the idea of fasting should be asked to do so. There are gentler ways, including mono-diets (see Chapter 5) which can start the process.

COMMON SIDE-EFFECTS OF FASTING

Awareness of the likely side-effects of fasting is important for both the person undertaking the fast and anyone supervising or looking after them. Such side-effects are usually relatively mild and are rarely serious, and include:

- Headaches (usually lasting less than a day, and common at the start of a fast). Nothing should be taken to suppress the headache. However, cold compresses, warm foot baths and neck massage should help (see Chapter 6).

- Insomnia is not uncommon at the start of a fast. Nothing should be taken to induce sleep. However, a neutral bath is often helpful as are the use of essential oils (see Chapter 6).

- Nausea and a coated tongue are usual on a fast, and if short-term fasting is repeated, as suggested in Chapter 5, these symptoms (and headaches) should steadily decrease in severity as detoxification becomes more established. Scraping the tongue and use of a herbal mouth-wash can help reduce these symptoms. The nausea will pass on its own. However, gentle acupressure on the 'anti-nausea' point on the wrist (see Chapter 6) should help minimize this symptom.

- Dizziness, light-headedness and palpitations are common early symptoms. They highlight the need for rest, and you should not drive or use machinery requiring strength or concentration during a fast. Relaxation and slow deep breathing exercises (see Chapter 6) are suggested to assist in the normalization of these transient symptoms. It is also suggested that during a fast you rise slowly from lying or sitting down, and that at the first sign of dizziness you lie down and rest. Dr Joel Fuhrman tells his male patients to sit during urination especially when rising to do so during the night.

- Increased body odour, skin rashes and dry skin may appear during a fast. Regular warm but not hot showers, or aromatherapy baths using appropriate oils (see Chapter 6) are suggested. The condition of the skin usually improves dramatically with regular short fasting. All such symptoms decrease as regular short fasts are undertaken.

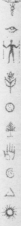

- Increased discharge from mucous membranes (nasal, vaginal, etc.) often occurs, and this should be allowed to happen unchecked during the fast.

- Aching limbs and muscles may occur early on in a fast (flu-like discomfort). Use of aromatherapy oils in a neutral bath, having a massage and doing light stretching exercises should ease these symptoms which reduce on their own as detoxification progresses.

- It is normal to feel colder than usual during a fast, and it is suggested that you dress more warmly than usual and add an extra blanket to the bed.

- As a rule hunger vanishes after the first day of a fast. Should it return this should be discussed with whoever is supervising the fast.

- Bed-rest is not essential or even desirable unless your physical condition demands it during a fast. Fresh air and a little gentle exercise are helpful, but excessive exercising (aerobic) and sunbathing should be avoided to conserve energy and prevent dehydration.

- The bowels may stop functioning during fasting, and this is not a concern. In long fasts, if there is a history of a toxic bowel, an enema or colonic irrigation may be suggested, although this is seldom necessary.

- If serious symptoms occur on a long fast, such as a sudden drop in blood pressure, or a feeling of extreme cold which persists, or a prolonged, rapid and weak pulse, or extreme weakness, or difficulty in breathing, then the fast should be stopped. These symptoms are extremely unlikely to occur on short fasts, but are possible on long-fasts, which highlights the need for supervision and the regular checking for vital signs.

- If vomiting and/or diarrhoea occur and are persistent, then expert advice should be sought. It is essential to maintain liquid intake at an optimum level, although this need not be excessively high (see Chapter 4).

- If acute anxiety and emotional distress are experienced then the fast should be broken. Be sure to very carefully follow the guidelines for breaking the fast (see Chapter 4) as this is a most important aspect of the whole procedure.

- If there are signs of hepatic or renal problems, the fast should be terminated.

- Uric acid levels in the bloodstream rise during a fast and, if there is a history of gout, caution is required. Ensure high levels of fluid intake (follow the guidelines in Chapter 4) to combat the development of gout during the fast, even if uric acid levels become relatively high.

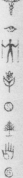

CLINICAL TESTS DURING LONG-TERM FASTING (MORE THAN FOUR DAYS)

- Salloum, Burton and Fuhrman (see particularly references 8 and 10 – from which many of the indications listed in this chapter are taken) as well as many other experts, suggest that during a supervised long fast there should be daily assessment of vital signs (heart, blood pressure, etc.) and weekly evaluation of electrolyte levels and reserves (which should be repeated if vomiting and/or diarrhoea or sudden weakness are noted).

- Before a long fast is started, suitable liver and kidney tests should be performed to evaluate the status of these vital organs. A long fast should be ruled out if the liver or kidneys are in a severely weakened or distressed state.

- Specific patterns of clinical results are unpredictable during a fast, as individual characteristics vary depending upon overall health status and any concurrent medical problems.

- Liver enzyme levels may rise, with or without liver disease being present.

- Cholesterol and triglyceride levels usually rise as fat stores are mobilized and uric acid levels rise (they should all fall after the fast).

- Blood glucose levels decline in most fasting individuals (and normalize subsequent to the fast).

- Erythrocyte sedimentation rate (ESR) usually decreases during a fast, while most aspects of a complete blood count remain stable if fluid intake is adequate.

- Increased specific gravity of urine usually indicates inadequate fluid intake. A variety of unusual products are commonly found in urine during a long fast.

- Insulin and thyroid hormone levels usually drop during a fast, while growth hormone increases (except in obese patients). Other increases usually include serum melatonin (assisting sleep and stress reduction), glucagon, cortisol, plasma norepinephrine.

- Blood pressure is likely to drop as is weight and pulse rate.

- As described later in the book, a marked improvement occurs in immune function, especially during the first 36 hours of a fast. There may be raised levels of T-lymphocytes and lymphokines, decreased complement factors, decreased antigen-antibody complexes, increased immunoglobulin levels, enhanced natural killer cell activity, heightened monocyte killing and bactericidal activity and a marked increase in resistance to infection in the post-fast period.

Despite this lengthy list of possible dangers and side-effects – fasting is safe, and short-term fasting is almost totally safe.

HOW TO FAST
(AND HOW
TO STOP FASTING)

I f you have never fasted before, and want to start to enjoy
some of the benefits of detoxification and regeneration, as
described in previous chapters, then you need to understand the essentials of fasting explained in this chapter.
Whether you are aiming to improve your health or to maintain
it, to retard the effects of ageing or to enhance detoxification,
there are a number of choices for you to make.

If, because of questionable health status with a history of
medication and health problems, you consider that the very real
benefits available from a long fast are what you need, then you
should consult someone trained and skilled in the use of fasting
and allied methods of health enhancement. Read the rest of the
book for greater awareness of what is involved, but essentially
you need to get advice and guidance before a fast is undertak-
en, and ideally an assurance of supervision when you do fast.

The information available in the Resources section at the end
of the book should assist you in finding this help.

Another choice would be to start to implement a series of
short fasts, or modified detoxification periods, as described
below.

Short fasts do work, but they take a good deal longer to produce the sort of benefits available from long fasts. They are

safer, however, especially if there is a history of drug use (medical or 'social') and/or exposure to and accumulation of toxic materials from food, industry or your environment.

LONG FAST OR SHORT FAST – WHEN DO YOU FEEL BENEFIT?

Whereas a long fast, of say 20 to 30 days in a residential clinic under expert supervision, might achieve marked health benefits, the same degree of improvement in health terms would take upwards of six months to a year of regular short-term fasting, two to three days at a time, once or (ideally) twice a month.

If less stringent detoxification methods, involving mono-dieting or modified fasting, were used instead of water-only fasting on these regular two to three day detoxification periods, then at least a year and probably longer would be needed to gain similar benefits – and this would only be achievable if the overall lifestyle and nutritional habits were modified to support the effort.

Before outlining what choices there are if short-fasts/detox periods are selected (see Chapter 5), and the ways in which both short and long fasts should be prepared for and undertaken (see below), it is useful to explain what is known about the physiology of our body's response to fasting.

WHAT HAPPENS ON A NORMAL TOTAL (WATER–ONLY) FAST?

There are three distinct stages of fasting as the body modifies its behaviour to conserve energy reserves, maintain a basic metabolic rate, and as it undertakes essential detoxification and repair strategies.

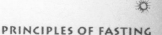

1) Early fasting

2) Fasting

3) Starvation

(Note: The third phase of fasting (starvation) will only occur if the true fast is not broken in time.)

1. **Early fasting**

During this stage, fuel for energy is derived from fat (adipose tissue), muscle tissue and enzymes present in the body. On the first day of any water-only fast, stores of glycogen in the liver are used up (within a matter of hours of the commencement of fasting) at which time much of the energy required to fuel the vital functions of the body is derived from fat stores in the form of fatty acids which are turned into energy in our body cells (in small 'factories' called mitochondria).

At this time glucose (sugar) is needed to supply the brain with energy, as well as to maintain blood sugar levels, because fatty acids cannot be processed by brain and blood cells in the same way as other body cells. For this reason, either glycerol deposits in the fatty tissues or amino acids found in muscle tissue are used as special energy sources for these areas of need. Both the kidneys and the liver are involved in the manufacture of energy from the various fuel sources as the fast progresses.

Were no other source of glucose available, we would break down and use up to 1 lb (450g) of muscle tissue daily to supply the glucose needs of the brain and bloodstream alone. However, after a few days of fasting (usually two days for females and three days for males) another source appears – ketones (a by-product of the breakdown of fats and proteins) which are manufactured in the liver, and which the body can turn into glucose for energy production.

It is at this time that toxic accumulations and fatty tissues begin to be removed from the body, and that homoeostasis becomes most effective in improving both physical and psychological health.

It is also the time when those individuals who have a history of prolonged or highly toxic medication and/or drug use, or whose health is compromised by other forms of toxic contamination (heavy metals, petrocarbons, pesticides, etc.) are most likely to be at risk if long-term fasting is undertaken without supervision.

During the first days of a fast, weight loss runs at around 2 lb daily, sometimes more. However, much of this is fluid which will be replaced. Over the length of a fast, average weight loss is approximately 1 lb (450g) daily.

2. Fasting

As the body forms ever increasing quantities of ketones, derived from the breakdown of fatty acids, these are used by the heart, blood and brain as sources of energy. However, the supply of ketones (acetoacetic acid, acetone and beta-hydroxybutyric acid) outstrips the ability of the body to utilize these acids as the fast progresses. To minimize the acidic build-up, bicarbonate which is present in the body is transformed into carbonic acid and then carbon-dioxide which is breathed out, so reducing the acid levels in the bloodstream. At this time the person fasting will probably notice that they are breathing more rapidly (as a means of eliminating more carbon dioxide) as well as their breath having a slightly unpleasant odour.

As early fasting changes to fasting proper (anywhere from the second to the fourth day of a fast, depending upon individual factors such as gender, body stores of fat, metabolic type and rate, health status, etc.) the body starts to adapt to the new situation and utilizes various strategies to conserve energy and recycle potential waste products.

During fasting proper, triglycerides are the main source of energy, derived from fatty tissues. At the same time, glucose is produced to fuel brain and blood requirements, from recycled lactic acid, a waste-product of muscular effort, and from recycled blood cells (in the liver), as well as from the steady breakdown of proteins (amino acids) taken from the muscles.

Naturopaths Salloum and Burton have reported on the research of many scientists, showing the ways in which the use of various sources of energy change, in an average weight individual, as a fast progresses.[1, 2, 3, 4]

In summary these are:

- Protein provides between 64g and 84g daily in early fasting, and this reduces to between 18g and 25g during fasting proper.

- Fat as a source of energy changes from between 100g and 140g to between 160g and 200g daily.

- Use of glucose alters from between 100g and 180g down to 80g daily.

- Sodium use moves from between 1.6g and 1.8g to between 0.02g and 0.035g daily.

- Potassium drops from 1.6g to 1.8g a day to 0.4g to 0.6g.

They also indicate the length of time various stores of energy would last were they the only sources available and if they were used up completely:

- Liver glucose stores are used up within an hour or so.

- Whatever food is being digested is used as an energy source and lasts for four to eight hours.

- Glycogen stored in the liver is used up over a period of about 12 hours.

- Amino acids which are freely available for energy use would last about 48 hours.

- Protein derived from muscles can fuel the body for about three weeks if it is used purely for manufacturing glucose, and for up to six months if only 'obligatory' use takes place while fat stores and ketones supply most energy.

- Triglycerides (fatty acids) in an average individual would last about two months as a fuel source.

3. Starvation
This starts when fat stores are completely utilized and the body has to turn to protein as its sole energy source, at which time vital tissues would be damaged, and death could result rapidly.

BEFORE YOU BEGIN

Before starting any detoxification programme, or a fast, you should ensure that it is appropriate to your needs and that you understand the do's and don'ts as listed below and in other chapters.

Even if you do not intend a lengthy fast, and wish to start to apply the suggested repetitive short fasts and/or detox options, as described in the next chapter, it would be wise to get professional advice to ensure that this is suitable to your current needs and health status. Consult the resources section to find a local practitioner or clinic (in many major cities there are naturopathic clinics attached to training colleges, which have modest fee structures).

The following questions and answers are meant to deal with most of the questions which first-time fasters ask.

Q. **How should I prepare for a fast?**

A. Follow the suggestions in the next chapter, in which cleansing and elimination are described, and try to prepare for the detoxification process of a fast by being in as healthy and 'clean' a state as possible.

On the day prior to a water-fast have light food only – fruits and salads ideally – with the 'last meal' before the fast being a very light one of, perhaps, just fruit.

Q. **How long should I fast?**

A. Why not try a weekend fast as described below. If begun on a Friday and ended on the Sunday evening a fast can last for 48 to 72 hours perfectly safely, without disrupting the normal flow of life, if you follow the guidelines as given, especially regarding breaking the fast. If you have an illness or condition which you believe requires a longer fast you should consult a suitably qualified practitioner for advice.

Q. **Should I exercise when I fast?**

A. You may feel energetic, but do not exercise apart from gentle stretching movements and a little walking, as energy is needed for the detoxification processes which are starting to take place. Rest and stay warm (being cold uses energy as well).

Q. **What 'symptoms' should I expect when I fast?**

A. You may feel colder than usual, so dress warmly.

You may develop a furred tongue and a bad taste in the mouth, so scrape your tongue and use a herbal or lemon-water mouthwash.

If a headache (or other symptoms such as nausea or muscle ache, as described above) develop, just rest, they will pass – do not take any medication to suppress these symptoms, if at all possible. A coffee enema (see Chapter 6) can often relieve nausea and a 'sick' headache by helping to flush the liver.

If you do feel that you have to take medication, break the fast first with a light snack (see below).

If you are at all distressed, and this is anything other than a short fast, get professional advice from whoever has agreed to supervise your fast.

In some instances a person may suffer 'withdrawal' symptoms if they have become addicted to certain foods or substances which are being avoided on the fast. These symptoms will pass, but if they are severe, get professional advice and consider gentler or more supervised fasting/detox with expert support (such as bodywork, acupuncture, homoeopathy, etc.) the next time.

Q. **Should I choose a water or a juice fast?**

A. A juice 'fast' is not really a fast at all but a restricted diet because there is an appreciable level of carbohydrate and other nutrients in juices which slows down (but does not completely stop) the biochemical changes which lead to ketosis in a water fast (see above). In water-only fasting the appetite usually vanishes, whereas on juice fasts hunger may remain. Certainly, weight loss is more sustained and pronounced on a water fast and there are some eliminative functions (of sodium, for example) which are more efficient.

Juice fasting, being less stringent, is far less likely to provoke any acute toxic reaction, which is possible, although rare, on a water fast.

Q. **How much should I drink on a fast?**

A. One of the leading experts on fasting, Trevor Salloum ND, suggests that most people should find a daily cup of water

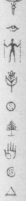

44   adequate, since the fat that is being transformed into energy and ketones releases a good deal of water.

While this may be true in healthy people who are fasting, I believe that a greater quantity is needed, especially as most experts agree that when a crisis does occur during a fast it is often because of dehydration and an excessive concentration of toxins.

If you are undertaking a water-only fast, then drink at least three pints of pure water (distilled, reverse osmosis purified or spring water – never chlorinated tap water) daily, and more if thirst calls for it, but not more than six pints (although some researchers suggest up to three litres daily for obese patients who are fasting). If you are on a juice or potassium broth detox-fast then follow the advice given in the instructions in Chapter 5.

Q. **Do I need to use an enema or have colonic irrigation during a fast?**

A. Probably not, but there may be times when, because of a particular bowel or other health problem, this is suggested. In which case take the professional advice you are given. Usually these treatments are not essential (especially on a water-only fast) despite a lot of emphasis placed on them by some schools of thought, most notably the German naturopathic/heilpraktiker approach. The coffee enema (described in Chapter 6) is, nevertheless, a useful means of assisting in clearing liver congestion (and associated feeling of nausea) and migraine headaches, and this can be used as described, if necessary.

On juice fasts, however, the need to flush the bowels may well arise if no bowel movements occur over a period of two or more days.

Q. **Can I chew gum to calm my hunger when I fast?**

A. Avoid chewing gum, because this stimulates your digestive system to start preparing for food. The objective of the fast is physiological rest, and an active but unsatisfied digestive system will both exhaust and confuse your body.

Q. **Do I need to take supplements during a fast?**

A. No, not unless you are taking the supplements L.acidophilus and/or bifidobacteria to help repopulate your intestinal tract's friendly bacterial flora, in which case these can be continued during a fast.

Some supplements inhibit the release of fatty acids from their storage sites, and most nutrients are well conserved by the body during fasting as part of its adaptation to 'famine' conditions, so supplementation is usually unnecessary.

Q. **Some experts recommend supplementing with a concentrated protein such as amino acid complex or spirulina during a fast. Is this a good idea?**

A. The only time such advice might be useful is in cases of extremely unstable hypoglycaemia (low blood sugar), which the fast should help correct anyway. If you are fasting on water, then take no supplements at all except for probiotics – friendly bacterial cultures (if these are already being taken). On detox programmes or during modified fasting (juice, broths, etc.), protein supplements are unnecessary.

Q. **What should I do if my sleep is disturbed during the fast?**

A. It is usual to sleep less deeply on a fast and, indeed, to have a very active mind. Try to relax, read, listen to pleasant music, and to do gentle stretching exercises, but take nothing to induce sleep. A 'neutral bath' (see Chapter 6) may help to relax you further.

Q. **What about a hot bath to relax me during a fast?**

A. As indicated, the fast is a period of physiological rest, and a hot bath would be enervating and potentially dehydrating (because it induces sweat). As mentioned, body-odour is likely to increase during a fast, and showers should be taken to

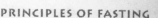

minimize the distress this might cause. Have neutral (tepid, body-heat) baths or showers, but not hot ones.

Q. **Will I be very hungry when I fast?**

A. Almost certainly not, especially after the first day. One of the most interesting phenomena associated with fasting is the complete absence of any desire for food once a fast is underway. It is a return of a clear tongue, sweet breath, boundless energy and a sharp mind, along with 'real' hunger that signals the time to break a long fast which has been successfully completed (symptoms should have disappeared as well!). This return of natural hunger can take anything from 10 to 30 days but, as stressed so many times in this book: only under supervision.

Q. **Should I continue working during a fast?**

A. No. It is best to rest. Do not under any circumstances drive a car or use complicated machinery during a fast.

Q. **Should I sunbathe during a fast?**

A. It is useful to get outdoors during a fast, for fresh air and indirect sunlight. Don't sunbathe for more than 15 minutes per day as any longer than this stresses the immune system.

Q. **What additional strategies should I adopt during a fast?**

A. Practise deep breathing, relaxation and meditation, as well as gentle (yoga-type) stretching.

Use skin brushing and neutral baths or showers to stimulate your skin's elimination functions, as well as to encourage a sense of calm, as described in Chapter 6.

Avoid the use of anti-perspirants during a fast, as these prevent normal elimination through the skin.

Use a coffee enema if you feel very nauseated or develop a migraine-type headache (see Chapter 6).

Q. **I am nervous about the whole idea of fasting, yet I understand its potential benefits. What should I do?**

A. Do not fast if you are at all nervous about the idea. Instead, try some of the gentler detox options listed in Chapter

5 and, as the benefits of these become apparent, try to talk to people who have fasted, get professional advice, read more about the subject, and then perhaps try some short 48 to 72 hour water-only fasts – if you feel ready for this.

Q. **How should I end a fast?**

A. This is a very important area and must be well understood before you start fasting.

More damage is done by breaking a fast wrongly than is ever caused by fasting itself.

Your stomach will have shrunk during a fast, and production of digestive enzymes will have all but ceased. The amount of food you can handle, as well as the amount needed to satisfy you, will be minimal at first, sometimes only a few mouthfuls of well chewed food (as described below) will suffice for a first meal.

Avoid anything spicy or heavily seasoned, and most certainly avoid eating meat during the first few meals after a fast.

The longer the fast, the more care is needed in its breaking. If possible, the first day after a full water-only fast of a week or more should involve no solid food, but diluted vegetable juice or a vegetable broth, sipped slowly and even 'chewed' (to ensure a good mix with the enzymes in the saliva).

Different experts have their own ideas as to how to break a fast safely, and some of these are listed below.

WHAT EXPERTS ADVISE FOR BREAKING A WATER-ONLY FAST

Dr Evarts Loomis MD[5] suggests that following a water-only fast, small, frequent, well-chewed meals are called for, with the first 'meal' comprising fruit or vegetable juice at breakfast, sipped slowly, followed by two to three more juices during the day. If the water fast has lasted more than one week, the juices should not be taken neat but diluted 50:50 with pure water.

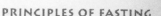

Water intake should be continued during these transition days. Loomis suggests that the juice days continue for two to three days after a one week water fast, and for four to five days if the water fast was longer than two weeks.

After these transition days, during which the dilution of the juices can gradually be reduced so that pure juice is being consumed by the third day, food intake should start as follows:

A breakfast of oatmeal soaked overnight with pineapple juice, with additional fresh fruit and a small amount of ground nuts. The other two meals of the first 'food' day should be of vegetables, raw or lightly cooked (steamed), after which a more normal eating pattern can be resumed.

The suggested pattern for breaking the fast from Dr Paavo Airola ND[6] is as follows:

> First day – eat a whole apple or other sweet fruit, chewing very well, and eating slowly. At the next meal have a bowl of fresh vegetable soup (unsalted and unspiced) or vegetable purée. On this day have your usual amount of water as well.

> Second day – the same as the previous day plus a glass of natural live low-fat yogurt.

> Third day – increase portions and add a raw side salad, some cooked rice and some natural cottage cheese.

> Fourth day – start to eat normally.

Dr James Balch MD[7] suggests that after a fast only raw foods should be eaten for the first two days, with the usual liquid intake maintained.

Dr Joel Fuhrman MD[8] suggests:

First day – fresh fruits and vegetables, with watermelon an ideal first meal on its own (a piece about the size of a fist is adequate). An option would be to eat an orange. One or the other of these should be eaten every two hours, with strict instructions to eat slowly and chew well. Another choice would be to start the process of eating again with fresh vegetable or fruit juice (as in Dr Loomis's suggestions above).

Second day – fruit or melon every three hours.

Third day – four meals comprising fruit meals, as before, and lettuce at the same time.

Fourth day – three meals to be eaten on this day, although these remain small, adding courgette (zucchini), tomatoes and cucumbers, plus a small amount of cooked vegetables such as potato or butternut squash.

Dr Fuhrman insists that over-ripe and under-ripe fruits should be avoided as they can cause abdominal cramp. He lists over-ripe pineapple as a particular danger. He also cautions against dry foods, such as nuts, baked potato, grains and dried fruit, as well as any spicy foods.

He is insistent that whole fruits are better than juices for breaking a fast because of their fibre content, which will encourage normal bowel function – although juice might be more helpful if potassium levels are low. A skilled expert in fasting should advise on what is best for you, as there are many considerations to be kept in mind when deciding what is best in any particular case.

Dr Boris Chaitow ND, DC[9] (who worked with Stanley Lief, his cousin, for many years) usually suggested to his patients

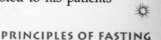

who had been fasting that they break their fast with a baked apple (no sweetening), or apple or pear purée. The recommended following meal was a small well-grated and shredded salad, and the one following that a lightly steamed vegetable meal with the emphasis on courgettes, squash, potato and carrots.

This is a pattern which I also promote, as well as sometimes suggesting a small bowl of vegetable soup, or a little (1 oz/28g or so) natural, low-fat, live yogurt or cottage cheese.

All these methods for breaking a fast refer to WATER-ONLY fasts. If a juice fast or mono-diet has been followed, then a great deal less care is needed in the transition back to normal eating. Guidelines will be given in the next chapter on what should be done when these detoxification or semi-fasts are carried out.

A SUMMARY OF WHAT TO EXPECT FOR FIRST-TIME FASTERS

Expect to feel unwell during the first day of your fast. You may suffer nausea, develop a headache, feel cold, perhaps feel a little dizzy and maybe experience palpitations. Certainly you will feel 'foggy-brained' and edgy, and there will be some muscle and joint aches. The important thing is to take nothing to suppress any of these symptoms while fasting.

If you fast for two days, expect to develop some nasal congestion, a mild skin rash and a degree of increased body odour. You will still feel cold and possibly dizzy, but by this time any headache and nausea will have eased.

Don't panic and don't despair. You are in the process of detoxification, and if there was no reaction at all you would be achieving very little indeed. Just rest, and use some of the measures described in Chapter 6 to make yourself more comfortable.

As detoxification takes place and your health improves, the mild discomfort felt during your first fast will dwindle, and future fasts will become pleasant experiences.

As time passes and fasts are repeated – especially if improvements are made in eating habits and lifestyle – your skin and eyes should become clearer, your brain sharper, your energy levels and your feeling of well-being distinctly better. But it takes time and will not happen after just one or two repetitions. It all depends on the level of toxicity present and the efficiency of your organs of detoxification – for instance, liver, kidneys, lungs and skin.

If you are at all unsure whether you should fast, seek advice from an expert (see the Resources list at the end of the book)

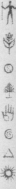

THE MANY WAYS
OF FASTING

I n this chapter details are given of a variety of fasting and detoxification methods, ranging from a supportive 'elimination' diet (which can also be used for identification of food allergy/sensitivity culprits) through variations on the theme of mono-diets and juice fasts (detoxification being their primary goal) to fasting proper, involving both short and long fasts. There are repeated reminders that anything over four days is regarded as a long fast which should never be undertaken without the approval and guidance of a health care professional knowledgeable in the use of fasting.

Before starting any detoxification diet or fast, pay some attention to organization and to the environment in which you will be spending time during this healing period.[1, 2, 3, 4, 5]

For example it is sensible to make sure that…

- …essential tasks are taken care of ahead of time.

- …people who care are aware of what you are doing and that they will be supportive and helpful should you need assistance (essential shopping, bills to be paid, pets to be cared for, etc.).

- ...you have adequate supplies of what you will need, most notably the fruit, or juice, or vegetable broth, or water that will be consumed, and that as much preparation is carried out ahead of time (washing, draining and wrapping fruit and vegetables to be juiced – and refrigerating these – for example).

- ...you have appropriate reading and audio material to amuse, inspire and relax you.

- ...you have important phone numbers to hand should you need to call for advice during the detox period/fast.

- ...you have fully understood what is called for on your part, and have the necessary foods for the ending of the detox period/fast ready, so that you do not have to start preparing food when you feel least like doing so.

Before a detox mono-diet, juice diet or fast it is wise to spend a few days on what can best be called a 'cleansing' diet.
This calls for the stopping of consumption of the following:

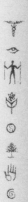

- Stimulant foods and drinks (don't drink anything but pure water, suggested (see below) herbal teas and fresh fruit/vegetable drinks).

- Refined and processed foods (no white flour products or sugar of any colour).

- High protein foods of animal origin (including eggs and most dairy produce, with the exception of virtually fat-free live yogurt or cottage cheese).

- Any fats of animal origin – and only cold-pressed vegetable oils (e.g. olive, flaxseed) and no heated fats or oils.

- In addition, pay attention to the quality of what you do eat – organic if possible and as fresh as you can get.

- If fruit or vegetables are not organic, remove the skin before eating or juicing, or your intake of toxic pesticides and fungicides and other sprays will increase.

ELIMINATION AND EXCLUSION DIETS

BORIS CHAITOW'S CLEANSING 'ELIMINATION' DIET[4]

This can last for one, two or more days, always preceding and if possible following a water-only or a juice fast for a day or so.

Ideally, before a fast proper at least one day should be spent on such a cleansing diet – longer if possible in order to minimize the initial toxic reaction which can produce a headache and nausea.

According to Boris Chaitow, the pattern as described can usefully be followed for between one and five days, both before and after a fast.

Breakfast

Choose one item from each of the following lists:

a) Apple, pear, 3–4 oz. (85–113g) grapes, peach, papaya (paw paw), mango, kiwi fruit, 3–4 oz. (85–113g) strawberries, blueberries, raspberries or other fresh berries in season, orange, grapefruit or other citrus fruit. Avoid avocado and banana at this meal.

b) 1–2 oz (28–57g) of sunflower or pumpkin seeds plus 1–2 oz (28–57g) of freshly-shelled walnuts, pecans, hazelnuts or almonds.

c) Drink either a cup of unsweetened herbal tea (safest teas are lemon balm, lime flower, linden blossom, raspberry leaf, lemon grass, fennel, anise, verbena, South African rooibos) or lemon juice in hot water.

Whatever herbal drinks you include, ensure also that not less than 4 pints (2 litres) of water are consumed throughout each day.

Main meals

At one of your main (mid-day/evening) meals choose from either of the following:

a) A mixed raw salad comprising not less than four varieties of salad vegetable which includes at least one orange/red item (beet, carrot, tomato, red pepper, etc.) as well as shredded green ingredients. Try to ensure that items such as celery, parsley and cress are regular ingredients for their mineral content.

b) Mixed stir-fried or steamed vegetables (ideal if digestion is sensitive to raw salads).

At one main meal, with either the salad (a) or the cooked vegetables (b) have one of the following:

a) A baked jacket potato (dressed with olive or flaxseed oil).

b) A cupful of boiled, unpolished rice or millet (cooked with a little onion for seasoning).

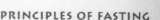

c) One or two bananas.

At the other main meal, choose one item from the following to accompany either salad or cooked vegetables:

d) An avocado pear.

e) 2 oz (57g) of cottage cheese (virtually fat free).

f) A poached or boiled egg.

g) Stir-fried or plain tofu (bean curd).

The idea of avoiding the mixing of concentrated carbohydrates and proteins at the same meal is based on the Hay Diet principle (known as 'food combining') – which remains unproven scientifically but is of obvious benefit to many people in enhancing their digestion and health. This calls for avoiding eating items (a), (b) or (c) at the same meal as items (d), (e), (f) or (g) – for example, no potato and cheese, and no egg and banana at the same meal.

Salad or cooked vegetable dressing: Cold-pressed virgin olive oil and lemon juice.

Dessert: Baked apple or pear purée.

TOM MOULE'S CLEANSING 'ELIMINATION' DIET[5]

Tom Moule ND was a widely respected naturopath who worked as assistant to Stanley Lief for many years and who became Director of Therapeutics at Champneys when Lief retired. The following is a detoxification diet recommended by Moule which he suggests could be conducted for up to 10 days every year.

I have made slight modifications to the description given by Tom Moule some 40 years ago, to take account of products no longer available.

Also, if the cleansing diet is being used to prepare for a fast, then the first three days described below should be ignored and only as many days as can be spared of the subsequent pattern of diet should be followed. Tom Moule describes a 10-day regime, the first three days on juice followed by a week of 'cleansing' diet:

> Early in the morning, on an empty stomach take an 8 fl oz (0.25 litre) glass of aperient water such as...one heaped teaspoon of Epsom salts and two teaspoons of Eno's or Andrews liver salts. The purpose of this is not merely to produce bowel function but to help in the elimination of acids and toxins from the blood-stream.

> For the remainder of the day take nothing but an 8 fl oz (0.25 litre) glass of fruit punch every three hours. Make the punch by squeezing two dozen oranges and one dozen lemons and add as much water as there is juice.

> Continue on this pattern for three days – the salts and water every morning and the fruit punch every three hours.

> At the end of the third day have a bowl of vegetable soup followed later by a fruit salad.

> For the remaining seven days of the detoxification regime follow the diet set out below:

> *On rising* – juice of a large lemon in a pint of water as hot as can be taken rapidly without discomfort.

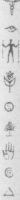

Morning meal – fresh fruit only (any kind other than bananas), as much as desired.

Mid-morning – cup of clear vegetable soup or fruit punch.

Mid-day – large raw vegetable salad with lemon juice and olive oil dressing, two to three slices of thin cold wholewheat toast or rice cake and butter. Fruit salad.

Mid-afternoon – fruit punch.

Evening – vegetable soup, salad, wholewheat bread, cheese.

Evening drink – clear vegetable soup or fruit punch.

This detoxification/cleansing diet, without the first three days of juice fasting, is an ideal pattern to prepare anyone for a subsequent fast, whether it is conducted for only a few days or the full week as suggested by Tom Moule.

ALLERGEN IDENTIFICATION USING EXCLUSION DIETS[6]

(I.E. FIVE-DAY FAST, OLIGOANTIGENIC EXCLUSION DIET, 'STONE-AGE' DIET, 'LAMB AND PEAR' DIET)

The oligoantigenic diet is not a fast, but because other aspects of allergen identification strategies (finding out what provokes an allergic reaction) are being explained, with the 'five-day fast' being the most stringent version of this, it is necessary for the sake of completeness to briefly outline the thinking behind the 'Stone-age diet', 'lamb and pear' diet and the oligoantigenic diet.

Many experts use versions of exclusion diets to help identify foods to which a patient is allergic or sensitive. By avoiding foods which may be provoking allergic symptoms for not less than five days (some experts say four days) all traces of any of the food will have cleared the system, and any symptoms caused by these should have vanished. Symptoms which remain are either caused by something else altogether (infection, for example) or by foods or other substances still in contact, internally or externally, with the individual.

On reintroduction of foods in a carefully controlled sequence (called a 'challenge') symptoms which reappear are shown to derive from a reaction to particular foods which are then eliminated from the diet for a considerable time.

The strictest of these exclusion diets is a **five day water-only fast** which is carried out under medical supervision, following which foods are carefully reintroduced to assess their impact on the production of symptoms. See the notes later in this chapter regarding short fasting methods for an understanding of what is involved.

The **'Stone-age diet'**[7] excludes those foods which have become a major part of human diet since Stone-age times, mainly grains of all sorts and dairy produce (in nomadic, hunter–gatherer societies there is no settled existence which would allow for growing crops or herding milk-producing animals). Also excluded on this diet are all modern processed foods involving any chemicals, colourings, flavourings, etc. Many Scandinavian researchers claim that a period on a Stone-age diet produces such benefits that a whole range of other allergies and health problems disappear.

The so-called **'lamb and pear' diet** is another fairly strict exclusion pattern, in which nothing is eaten except for lamb (including various organs and offal), pears with their skins and bottled mineral water. The reason for the selection of these two foods is that very few people are allergic to either of them. The diet is infinitely boring and stressful (and impossible for people

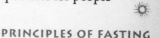

of a vegetarian disposition). It is, however, easier for many people to follow than a water fast.

The **oligoantigenic diet** consists of a far fuller eating pattern, and is derived from many years of research at Great Ormond Street's Hospital for Sick Children in London, and at Addenbrookes Hospital in Cambridge. The oligoantigenic diet is usually followed for up to three weeks while symptoms are evaluated. If they vanish, then one or more of the foods being avoided may be to blame. Identification and subsequent avoidance of the culprit food(s) depends upon the symptom returning upon the reintroduction (challenge) of the food.

The eating pattern is listed below and has been found very helpful in identification of the allergens which can trigger eczema, recurrent ear infections, asthma, bedwetting, hyperactivity and bowel problems, especially in children.

Meats

Allowed: Lamb, turkey, rabbit, game (lean and cooked plainly).

Forbidden: Beef, chicken, pork, preserved meats, bacon, sausages.

Fish

Allowed: White fish (not if eczema present).

Forbidden: All smoked fish, shellfish.

Vegetables

Allowed: All except those forbidden – patients with bowel problems are asked to avoid beans, lentils, brussels sprouts and cabbage.

Forbidden: Potatoes, tomatoes, onions, soya and sweetcorn.

Fruit

Allowed: Bananas, peeled pears, pomegranates, paw-paw, mango.

Forbidden: All fruits except the five allowed ones.

Cereals

Allowed: Rice, sago, millet, buckwheat.

Forbidden: Wheat, oats, rye, barley, corn.

Oils

Allowed: Sunflower, safflower, linseed, olive.

Forbidden: Corn, soya, 'vegetable', nut (especially peanut).

Dairy

Allowed: None (Tomor and Vitasieg margarine are allowed).

Forbidden: Cow's milk and all its products including yogurt, butter, most margarines, all goat, sheep and soya milk products, eggs.

Drinks

Allowed: Some herbal teas such as chamomile and those listed above as the allowed drinks during the 'cleansing' diet plus pure water.

Forbidden: Tea, coffee, fruit squashes, citrus drinks, apple juice, alcohol, tapwater, carbonated drinks.

Miscellaneous

Allowed: Sea salt.

Forbidden: Yeast products, chocolate, preservatives, all food additives, herbs, spices, honey, sugar of any sort.

To make sense of what is happening on any exclusion diet professional advice is needed. Several (up to three) weeks on a 'Stone-age', 'lamb and pear' or oligoantigenic diet might dramatically improve a wide range of symptoms resulting from allergy. Identifying what those foods are which provide allergic reactions requires patience and, usually, professional help.

MONO-DIETS

By definition, a mono-diet is one in which only a single food is eaten for a period. Probably the most famous is the 'grape cure' which has been used for many years as a means of treating chronic disease.

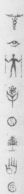

Note: If you do embark upon a mono-diet, then ensure that the food you choose is organically grown, unsprayed and free of all chemical preservatives.

An **apple** mono-diet is suggested for acidic conditions such as gout and inflammation. Eat the skin as well since you will have chosen organically grown fruit.

Grapes – especially black ones – are suggested for cardiac conditions, arthritis and blood pressure problems (grapes are potassium-rich). Again, the chosen grapes will be organically grown (if they are not, then do not start a mono-diet), so eat the skins (and pips) as well.

Pears are ideal for allergy sufferers (eat the skins as well).

A **grapefruit** mono-diet is recommended for liver conditions, while an **orange** mono-diet is suggested for a catarrhal condition.

Papaya and carrot mono-diets are suggested for people with digestive problems.

Whole (brown) rice mono-diets are recommended for high blood pressure and as an excellent detoxification method.

A mono-diet involves eating just one food of your choice for up to four days. As a rule, if a longer period is needed, then, just as with fasting, professional advice and possibly supervision should be sought.

On mono-diet days drink not less than 3 pints (1.75 litres) of water, and not more than 6 pints (3.5 litres). Drink a little whenever thirsty. Too little water may induce constipation.

Anyone with an active yeast problem, such as thrush or candidiasis, should avoid fruit mono-diet choices until the yeast is controlled.

QUANTITIES OF FOOD ON MONO-DIET DAYS

On each day of the mono-diet, not more than 3 lb (1.5kg) weight of the selected fruit should be eaten, in small amounts, throughout the day.

Paavo Airola[8], in describing a two-week grape diet, has the patient eat no more than a few grapes at breakfast and lunch on the first day and a few ounces in the evening. On the second day he suggests several ounces at each meal, with a gradual increase in quantity so that by the fourth day as much as is desired is eaten – grapes only, of course – with an upper limit of 3–4 lb (1.5–2kg) daily.

If unprocessed (whole) rice or other grains (buckwheat, millet, for example) are selected for a mono-diet, then 1 lb (0.5kg) dry weight (i.e. before cooking) of an organically grown variety should be the maximum per day.

This should be cooked conservatively by placing the washed rice (or other grain) in a saucepan and covering with water. Bring to the boil and simmer until soft (all the water having been absorbed). If allowed to stand for 10 minutes it will be ready to eat.

When the rice/grain has cooled it should be divided into servings (five or six servings out of this quantity since each measure of rice becomes three measures once cooked) and, before eating, add to each serving a half-dessertspoonful of olive oil and the juice of one lemon (some people add tamari sauce).

Cooked rice and grains remain palatable and safe to eat for up to five days if kept in a cool dry place.

THE MODIFIED FAST

(JUICE OR 'POTASSIUM BROTH')

As indicated, a juice fast is not a fast at all but a detoxification diet, a 'modified' fast, and as such it is a very powerful tool in any attempt at recovering health, regenerating the functions and organs of the body, boosting immune response and as a supportive tactic to pure-water fasting, before and/or after use of this ultimate healing method.

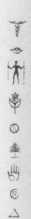

I present several versions of the modified fast as this is probably the most attractive option for anyone new to the idea of fasting, for whom water-only fasting may seem extreme and something to try a little later on.

The benefits of modified fasting are exactly the same as those of water-only fasting, only it takes a lot longer to achieve the major benefits by this method.

ENEMAS – YES OR NO?

The use of enemas before, during or after modified and water-only fasting is a hotly debated subject. In the methods which are described below, those of Moule, Rauch and Airola all suggest enemas. However, they are at variance with the views of Salloum and Burton[9], who clearly state: 'Enemas are not usually necessary and may not offer any added benefit. Some authorities have found that they cause discomfort. To help prevent constipation a pre-fast meal of fresh fruit or vegetables will assist elimination.'

As explained in Chapter 1, my personal experience as a child may have coloured my judgement as to the virtues of enemas. They can be necessary, especially on a mono-diet or juice/vegetable broth elimination diet, if the bowels fail to move after several days. However, I agree with Salloum and Burton's statement that they are seldom needed on a regular water-only fast.

The use of coffee enemas, as described in Chapter 6, for symptomatic treatment of nausea/migraine headache, have a completely different objective from that of a water enema – i.e. the flushing of bile from the liver rather than the clearance of the lower bowel. Coffee enemas are recommended when such symptoms appear, especially on a long water-only fast.

In cases of bowel toxaemia (dysbiosis) I sometimes suggest colonic irrigation, which is a more complete flushing of the entire colon. However, this is also totally dependent upon individual needs and is not regularly prescribed.

A variety of modified fasts are presented below to help illustrate both the differences and the similarities of these detoxification methods. Selection of one as opposed to another may well be a matter of personal preference, since there are no studies to show whether one is more effective than another. All have their supporters, all have detoxification and regeneration potential, and all are potentially health enhancing.

THE LIEF/MOULE 'SHORT' MODIFIED FAST

This version of a modified fast was described in a Champneys handbook published in 1962, the year before Stanley Lief's death, at which time Tom Moule ND was Director of Therapeutics at the famous Tring health resort.[5]

This fast should not exceed three days (72 hours) without supervision.

> On rising in the morning, take no food, but have a drink of hot water, to which a little lemon may be added, if desired. Every two hours throughout the day, from 8 am until 8 pm, take approximately a half cup of carrot juice, apple juice or clear vegetable soup. It is important that nothing else should be taken, otherwise the total value of the fast will be lost entirely.

If there should be a slight fever it is desirable to drink more water.

After three days...

> ...the fast should be broken by taking a little natural [low fat] yogurt, every two hours, but nothing else on that day except water.

'On the following two days, the following diet should be taken after which a normal pattern may be resumed:

Breakfast – Half a cup of carrot juice or apple juice or clear vegetable soup.

Mid-day – Varied raw salad and two portions of crispbread and butter.

Evening – One steamed green vegetable with steamed carrots and a vegetarian savoury flavouring. Stewed prunes, raisins and other fruit may be eaten afterwards.

As indicated above, Tom Moule had firm ideas about the use of enemas during fasting, and these are described in Chapter 6.

DR ERICH RAUCH'S TEA FAST[10]

Erich Rauch MD heads a large health spa in Austria, and his suggested 'tea fast' represents an approach in the early treatment of infection, when fasting can be the most valuable of methods for boosting immune function.

Dr Rauch suggests that, as a treatment for colds and infection, nothing should be eaten in the early and acute stages – until such symptoms as fever, shivering, headache, nausea and vomiting have subsided.

If shivering is a symptom, the liquids should be hot; and if feverish, they should be cool, but not ice-cold.

The teas suggested are:

- Linden (lime) flower and lilac, which both induce perspiration if taken hot.

- Rose-hip tea, which is vitamin C rich and promotes kidney function. This should be consumed cold.

- Chamomile tea which is calming and which helps digestive symptoms.

Dr Rauch suggests the addition of a little (a teaspoon of each) honey and lemon juice or buckthorn juice to the tea.

Other teas which might prove useful are:

- Elder flower, which loosens phlegm and induces sweat.

- Mullein, for loosening phlegm and alleviating coughs.

- Peppermint, which helps stomach symptoms, clears breathing and has a stimulant action.

- A 'basic catarrh tea' can be made from a mixture of 1 oz (28g) each of plantain and coltsfoot, plus 0.7 oz (20g) each of licorice and horsetail. These are mixed, and a tea is prepared from the resulting combination.

No schedule is given by Dr Rauch for consumption of teas, but his instructions are clear on how long this regime should continue:

Unless otherwise directed you should begin a tea fast immediately, either in the preliminary stages or at the outbreak of illness [infection]. No food is to be taken...but herb tea is to be drunk frequently and copiously. When the disease has been conquered and continuing strong hunger is felt, fasting can gradually be discontinued.

See Chapter 6 for Dr Rauch's views on the use of enemas during a fast and during infection.

PAAVO AIROLA'S JUICE OR BROTH FAST[8]

Dr Airola based his fasting technique on that of many experts. In particular he quotes the work of Dr Otto Buchinger Jr, whom he describes as 'the champion of therapeutic fasting in modern times' (Airola was writing in the 1970s).

Dr Airola uses Buchinger's arguments to support the choice of 'juice and broth' fasts over plain water fasting, when he states:

Raw juices, as well as freshly made vegetable broths, are rich in vitamins, minerals, trace elements and enzymes. These are easily assimilated directly into the bloodstream with no strain on the digestive system. They are extremely beneficial in…supplying needed elements for the body's own healing activity, thus speeding recovery. Raw juices and vegetable broths provide an alkaline surplus which is extremely important for the proper acid-alkaline balance, since blood and tissues contain large amounts of acids during fasting.

Airola suggests that on the day before the proposed fast the bowels be cleared by a combination of castor oil dosage and enemas.

On the day of the commencement of fasting:

On rising – Cup of lukewarm herbal tea (peppermint, chamomile, red clover, rose hip are suggested)

9–10 am – Glass of freshly prepared juice (orange, apple, grape, pear) diluted 50:50 with pure water (no canned or frozen juices should be used).

1 pm – Glass of fresh vegetable juice (carrot, celery, tomato) diluted with water, or a glass of vegetable broth (see Airola's recipe below).

4 pm – Cup of herbal tea.
7 pm – Glass of vegetable or fruit juice diluted with water.
9 pm – Chamomile enema.

In addition, plain lukewarm water can be consumed when thirsty. The total volume of juice consumed during 24 hours should be between 1.5 pints (0.9 litre) and 1.5 quarts (1.7 litres).

The fast is broken with one item of fruit and one bowl of vegetable soup or purée, as well as the usual juices and broth for one day.

VEGETABLE BROTH RECIPE
2 large potatoes chopped or sliced
1 cup carrots, shredded or sliced
1 cup celery, chopped or shredded, leaves and all
1 cup of any other available vegetable, such as beet tops,
turnip tops, parsley or a little of each of these
(Paavo Airola reminds us that the broth can be made with just the potatoes, carrots and celery.)

The ingredients are put into a stainless steel saucepan and covered with 1.5 quarts (1.7 litres) of water, brought to the boil and simmered for 30 minutes. The liquid is then strained from the vegetables, and allowed to cool until warm, when it is ready to serve. If not used immediately, the broth should be kept in a refrigerator and warmed before use.

JOHN LUST'S JUICE FAST[11]
In promoting his juice fast, John Lust contends that, as a means of 'cleansing', fruit juices are preferable to vegetable juices which he regards as 'regenerators and builders' of the body. His fast calls for several days on juice (and water) alone as a precursor to a tailored dietary regime for specific conditions.

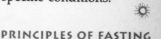

He has listed particular juices for a host of conditions, some of which are summarized below.

John Lust suggests drinking no more than 16 fl oz (0.5 litre) of juice daily, sipped slowly in small amounts each time, with water added as required. Some juices, he states, are too 'potent' to be used on their own, and these should be diluted with other juices, usually carrot.

The potent juices are: beet, beet greens, spinach, parsley, dandelion, garlic, asparagus, lemon (dilute this with water), watercress and turnip.

The following are John Lust's recommendations for particular conditions (two days maximum of 16 fl oz/0.5 litre of juice mixtures daily, plus water):

Acne

16 fl oz (450ml) of carrot alone, or 10 fl oz (285ml) carrot and 6 fl oz (170ml) spinach.

Allergies/Arthritis/Asthma

6 fl oz (170ml) carrot, 5 fl oz (142 ml) beet and 5 fl oz (142ml) cucumber, or 8 fl oz (230ml) carrot and 8 fl oz (230ml) celery.

Colitis

8 fl oz (230ml) carrot and 8 fl oz (230ml) apple.

Constipation

8 fl oz (230ml) carrot, 4 fl oz (110ml) celery and 4 fl oz (110ml) apple.

Diarrhoea

6 fl oz (170ml) carrot, 6 fl oz (170ml) celery and 2 fl oz (55ml) parsley.

Gastric ulcer

8 fl oz (230ml) carrot, 4 fl oz (110ml) cabbage and 4 fl oz (110ml) celery.

Note: Under controlled supervised conditions at Stanford University, a quart (1 litre) of cabbage juice (cabbage is rich in vitamin U, as is celery) was taken in five separate 6 fl oz (170ml)

doses, added to the diet of people with gastric ulceration. X-ray
pictures showed remarkable healing results.

Hay fever

6 fl oz (170ml) carrot, 5 fl oz (142ml) beet and 6 fl oz (170ml) cucumber.

Headaches

8 fl oz (230ml) carrot, 5 fl oz (142ml) and 3 fl oz (85ml) spinach.

Heart problems

7 fl oz (200ml) carrot, 4 fl oz (110ml) celery, 2 fl oz (55ml) parsley and 3 fl oz (85ml) spinach.

Heartburn

8 fl oz (230ml) carrot and 8 fl oz (230ml) apple.

Haemorrhoids

8 fl oz (230ml) carrot and 8 fl oz (230ml) watercress.

Insomnia

10 fl oz (285ml) carrot and 6 fl oz (170ml) celery.

Jaundice

Juice of half a lemon in warm water in the morning followed by 10 fl oz (285ml) carrot juice.

Liver problems

11 fl oz (312ml) carrot, 3 fl oz (85ml) beet and 2 fl oz (55ml) coconut.

Migraine

10 fl oz (285ml) carrot and 6 fl oz (170ml) spinach.

Nervous system

8 fl oz (230ml) carrot and 8 fl oz (230ml) celery.

Rheumatism

6 fl oz (170ml) carrot, 5 fl oz (142ml) beet and 5 fl oz (142ml) celery.

Sinus problems

Juice of a whole lemon and 4 fl oz (110ml) of ground (not pressed) horseradish, or 10 fl oz (285ml) carrot, 3 oz (85ml) beet and 3 oz (85ml) cucumber.

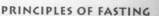

8 fl oz (230ml) carrot and 8 fl oz (230ml) pineapple, or 8 fl oz (230ml) carrot and 8 fl oz (230ml) celery.

Note: The same rules regarding supervision apply to juice and broth fasts as to water-only fasts.

No more than three days (72 hours) should be spent on the fast without supervision, and even for this short period, if you are not already experienced in these methods, it is wise to first discuss your need for a fast, the protocols of fasting and, most important, how to break the fast, with a suitably qualified health care professional.

DR EVARTS LOOMIS'S JUICE FAST[12]

After years of water-only fasts, Dr Loomis modified his approach, having become impressed by the effectiveness of the Swiss-based Landhaus Nurpfli Retreat and the Bircher-Benner Clinic juice-fasting methods which he found to be more effective in many ways, and which also, unlike water fasting, created a pattern which was more likely to be maintained after the fast was broken.

Dr Loomis commonly precedes a fast by having the patient go onto a 'transition diet' which comprises grains and steamed vegetables. He also suggests starting a fast with three nightly enemas and liver flushes (see below). A teaspoon of vitamin C powder compounded with potassium, sodium, magnesium and calcium is added to the enema solution. A bowel purge using a laxative such as sodium phosphate is also administered.

During a fast, carrot and green vegetable juice combinations (50:50) are suggested by Dr Loomis, as well as herbal teas and the consuming of a broth named after the famous medical naturopath Henry Bieler MD.

'Bieler broth' is made by steaming green beans, courgettes [zucchini], celery and parsley. These are then puréed and eaten with a spoon in small quantities during the 'modified fast'.

Before and during the fast, if detoxification is considered necessary, Dr Loomis adds a special bedtime cocktail consisting of a blend of a clove of garlic, juice of half a lemon, juice of two grapefruits (or apple juice) plus two tablespoons of olive oil.

This 'liver-flush' is aimed at detoxifying that essential organ – something also achieved by use of a coffee enema according to many experts (see Chapter 6).

The length of a fast is related to each patient's needs and response to treatment, and the outlines of Dr Loomis's fasting methods, given here, are not meant to be taken as a prescription. They are provided to illustrate the many variations that exist in juice/modified fasting. Dr Loomis's patients commonly fast for several weeks using his approach.

AYURVEDIC SHORT FAST[13]

Traditional Indian medicine (Ayurveda) includes fasting as a major part of its methodology. Writing on the subject, Scott Gerson MD states:

> Fasting on one day a week is recommended for the normal healthy individual. It is an effective initial treatment for many diseases because it rids the body of toxins, and enlivens…the digestion…many variations of fasts are described in Ayurveda, ranging from the time-honoured water fasts to fasts incorporating various juices, teas and broths. Before undertaking a fast of any duration it is highly advisable to seek the advice of an Ayurvedic physician or other qualified practitioner.

> The amount of liquid taken varies, but in general one should take between 2 and 4 pints [1 and 2 litres] each day. Fruit juices are discouraged…although certain herbs if taken in the form of tea during the fast will assist in elimination of toxins from the body.

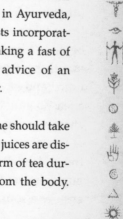

These include black pepper, long pepper, cayenne, dry ginger, asafoetida, basil and cardamom.

DR MAYR'S 'DRY' FAST[14, 15]

The famous Austrian physician Franz Xavier Mayr focused much of his healing work on improving the digestive systems of his patients. He came to believe that to simply alter a person's dietary pattern was less than half of the required change needed to restore health, and that equally – or even more important – was the need to restore health to the digestive system. In attempting to achieve this he evolved a highly successful, complex dietary/modified fasting regime ('The Mayr Cure') which is widely followed in Germany and Austria, and increasingly in other countries of Europe as its efficacy becomes more well known.

The modified version presented below is suitable for home application, and differs from the methods which would be more stringently applied in a clinic using the 'cure'.

THE TWO-WEEK (MODIFIED) MAYR CURE

For breakfast, slowly chew a stale (three day old) dry, white roll (or one which has been dried in a warm oven) with no liquid being taken at all during the meal. Each small mouthful should be chewed not less than 40 times, until the contents of the mouth become a smooth paste. When you have chewed 40 times, and have the now liquidized mouthful of dry roll, place a teaspoonful of plain low-fat live yogurt into your mouth and chew a few more times and then swallow.

This chewing stimulates the centre in the brain (satiety centre) which tells you when you have eaten enough, it also thoroughly mixes the roll with ptyalin enzymes in your saliva, and ensures a sound digestion of the food.

During breakfast you will eat approximately a quarter of a tub of live-yogurt and a stale roll. Nothing should be taken apart from these two foods.

Half an hour after this meal, drink a herbal tea (choose from fennel, sage, lemon verbena, linden (lime) blossom, chamomile, peppermint).

For lunch and your evening meal, go through precisely the same process with a dry roll and yogurt as you did at breakfast. Then have a variety of cooked vegetables (steamed or stir-fried, for preference) together with a little (2 oz/57g maximum) fish or tofu, if this is desired.

Half an hour after each meal have a herbal tea.

During the day sip water when thirsty.

During the two weeks of the diet ('cure') you can carry on working as normal (but allow more time than usual for meals as the roll takes time to chew through!).

Throughout these two weeks eat no fruit or raw vegetables, and no fatty foods. Have no alcohol or coffee, and absolutely no sugar.

This programme helps to regenerate the digestive system.

Note: The Mayr Cure echoes another famous 'dry fasting' method, the Schroth Cure which was for many years successfully used in Germany and some UK health resorts to treat seriously ill patients with chronic degenerative diseases. The Schroth diet also included dry rolls or rusks as one of its methods of encouraging healing. To my knowledge this is no longer available in the UK as the skills required for its application seem to have vanished along with the time required for people to devote to its stringent requirements.

THE SCHROTH CURE DIET[16]

According to one of Britain's leading naturopaths, Roger Newman Turner, the Schroth Cure was meant to offer a strong stimulus to the metabolism and to promote skin elimination. The diet calls for alternate 'dry' and 'wet' days (see below) and for the application of various associated hydrotherapy measures (cold packs in particular) to enhance skin activity.

(The wet or cold pack is one in which damp cotton material is wrapped around an area (trunk, limb, etc.) and covered with an insulating layer of (usually) woollen blanket, which allows it to heat up (using body heat) and eventually bake dry. In the USA this sort of treatment is more accurately called a 'warming compress'.)

Roger Newman Turner describes a typical Schroth regime as follows:

First day – Dry toast or semi-stale rolls until mid-day. Oatmeal or rice porridge.

4pm onwards – 4 fl oz (100ml) warm dry wine or apple juice. Rice or barley gruel. A cold ('warming') pack at night.

Second day – Toast or dry biscuits until mid-day. Porridge with apple sauce.

4pm onwards – 1 pint (500ml) herbal tea, fruit juice or wine. Cold pack.

Third day – Toast, dried prunes or baked jacket potato. Lemon slices if very thirsty.

The cycle is repeated for a period of two to three weeks.

The main application of this method was in the treatment of chronic skin conditions, catarrhal states and chronic diseases such as rheumatoid arthritis – for which successful results were often claimed.

Dr Haas, Director of Marin Clinic of Preventive Medicine and Health Education in California, has developed a detoxification and regeneration diet which he suggests be followed for anything up to four weeks. His diet aims at eliminating those foods which encourage the accumulation of acid wastes. Dr Haas cautions that for the first few days you may feel off-colour (as in most detox programmes) but that by the third or fourth day…'clarity and a feeling of well-being should appear.'

Among his basic suggestions are:

- Chewing very well – 30 to 50 chews per mouthful.

- Relaxing before each meal (see Chapter 6).

- Sitting comfortably when eating.

- Eating mainly of steamed fresh vegetables and greens.

- Drinking nothing apart from herbal teas after meals.

- Eating nothing after 6.30 pm.

HAAS'S DETOX MENU

On rising – Two glasses of water (reverse osmosis, spring or filtered), one of which is mixed with the juice of half a lemon.

Following some stretching exercises, have one serving of a fresh fruit. (Choose from banana, apple, pear, grapes or citrus.) Between 15 and 30 minutes later, eat one bowl of cooked whole grains (chosen from millet, brown rice, amaranth or quinoa [South American cereals], or buckwheat). Flavour this with two teaspoons of fruit juice.

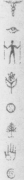

Lunch (noon to 1.00 pm) and *evening meal* (5.00 to 6.00 pm) – These should comprise one to two medium-sized bowls of steamed vegetables using a variety of root, stem and leaf vegetables. Remember Dr Haas's 'chewing' guidelines.

Dr Haas suggests as 'seasoning' a mixture of cold-pressed canola oil and regular butter – no more than one teaspoon per meal. (Author's note: Virgin cold-pressed olive oil or flaxseed oil – a teaspoon per meal on vegetables – would serve the same purpose.)

Mid-morning and mid-afternoon (11.00 am and 3.00 pm) – Drink one to two cups of vegetable water, saved from the steamed vegetable cooking process. A little sea salt or kelp can be added. Each mouthful should be kept in the mouth and be well mixed with saliva before swallowing.

During the evening – Herbal teas such as peppermint, Pau D'arco or chamomile can be drunk.

THE WAERLAND'S ALKALINE-DETOX DIET[18]

The famous Swedish nutritional experts, Are and Ebba Waerland, have designed their own version of an alkaline broth, the consumption which has as its objectives the neutralization of acid wastes, the encouragement of elimination of toxic materials and the normalization of peristaltic bowel action – so avoiding the need for enemas.

The drink which accomplishes all of these ideals is called 'Excelsior'. It is prepared in the evening for use the next day and is kept refrigerated and warmed to body heat before drinking it, without any chewing.

Before describing how to make 'Excelsior' it is necessary to place it in the context of the overall detoxification and health enhancement programme which the Waerlands advocate, which although conceived as being largely a preventive approach, rather than a treatment protocol, in practice is usually undertaken with great benefit by people who are already ill.

The programme calls for the following protocol:

On waking – One to two cups of 'Excelsior'. Morning neck and head massage, a cold shower, a dry-brush massage (see Chapter 6), morning exercises or a brisk walk.

Breakfast – Yogurt, fresh fruit.

Between meals – Herbal teas.

Lunch – Cooked or uncooked grain meal, 'kruska' (see recipe below), plus stewed fruit and, if desired, wholemeal bread, mild cheese, onions).

Evening meal – Large salad, including beets, carrots and onion, plus any green salad vegetables – baked or boiled unpeeled organic potatoes, plus sour-dough rye bread, butter and cottage cheese.

The Waerland system calls for the avoidance of salt, vinegar, pepper, mustard, strong spices, coffee, tea, tobacco, alcohol, white sugar or white flour products, canned or processed foods, meat, fish or eggs.

'EXCELSIOR'

One cup of vegetable broth (see recipe in Paavo Airola's Juice or Broth Fast)

1 tablespoon of flaxseed (linseed)

1 tablespoon of wheat bran

The flaxseed and wheat bran are soaked overnight in the vegetable broth (refrigerated), and in the morning the drink is warmed to body heat, well stirred and drunk without any chewing, seeds and all. This drink is a superb conditioner of the digestive system, since it enhances peristaltic action naturally without any irritation. If it is used on a fast (no solids) then it should be strained before being consumed.

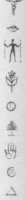

RECIPE FOR WAERLAND'S 'KRUSKA' CEREAL

A tablespoon each of organic whole wheat, whole rye, whole oats, whole barley, whole millet

2 tablespoons each of wheat bran and unsulphured raisins

The grains should be ground coarsely and placed in a pot with 1.5 cups of water, and the bran and raisins should then be added. This is boiled for five to 10 minutes. The pot is then wrapped in a blanket or newspapers and allowed to stand for several hours. If the resulting porridge is mushy, use less water next time. Serve this hot with yogurt or homemade apple purée or stewed fruit (no sugar).

Exactly the same ingredients can be used without cooking by pouring boiling water over the ground grains and other ingredients, allowing this to steep for half an hour before serving as described above. This 'uncooked' method retains enzymes and vitamins, but is slightly more difficult to digest and should not be used by anyone with an irritable bowel problem.

THE GUELPA FAST[19]

The Guelpa fast involves the use of salts such as Epsom salts to promote detoxification, especially in rheumatic conditions.

The day is started with a teaspoon of Epsom salts in warm water, and for the rest of the day only warm water containing a slice of lemon and a little honey, or a vegetable (potassium) broth, should be consumed.

Epsom salts start the next day as well, followed by fruit juices throughout the day, and vegetable soup and dry wholemeal toast at night.

On the third day, dry biscuits or toast, and possibly a baked potato, are eaten during the day, but with no fluids at all being allowed until 6 pm, at which time a glass of dry white wine is taken as it is again at 9 pm.

After these three days the patient is asked to spend a few days on salad, fruit and yogurt.

There are clear similarities between elements of the Schroth, Guelpa, Lief/Moule, Loomis, Haas, Waerland, Mayr and other fasting programmes and each has its supporters and detractors. All of them achieve detoxification, but none is as effective at regeneration and detoxification as the 'real thing' – the water-only fast.

SHORT WATER-ONLY FAST

Unlike modified fasting using juices and/or broth, which have as their main aim detoxification, plus some of the benefits of water fasting (albeit achieved in a slower manner), water-only fasts have particular objectives and effects.

- There is a 'physiological rest' period during which time detoxification, repair and regeneration are accelerated.

- Immune function is boosted and auto-immune conditions are helped.

- Growth hormone production from the pituitary gland is stimulated, with marked anti-ageing and repair benefits.

Bearing in mind the contraindications described in the previous chapter, the following is my protocol for a short (maximum 72 hours) water-only fast:

On the evening before the first day of the fast, having eaten lightly throughout the day, have a fruit-only salad or natural yogurt snack, and nothing else at all except water as desired.

On waking, have a tumbler of warm water and a touch (a few drops for taste only) of lemon juice, sipped slowly.

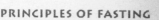

Spend the day resting, reading, listening to restful music, with intermissions of stretching, deep breathing and relaxation, both indoors and out.

Have an 8 fl oz (230ml) tumbler of water, hot or cold, with or without a touch of lemon, every two hours at least, sipped slowly.

Throughout the day, consume not less than 4 pints (2 litres) and not more than 8 pints (4 litres) of water.

Be prepared to feel restless and colder than usual, with odd symptoms as described in earlier chapters. You may find that you cat-nap but cannot sleep for lengthy periods. This is normal. Take nothing to alter the 'symptoms' of fasting as these indicate that the process is under way and normal. Dress more warmly than usual, rinse your mouth and/or clean your teeth, stretch and do some deep breathing, or take a neutral bath or shower. Get a massage if possible.

These are the best and safest ways of modifying your symptoms. Do not be concerned if your bowels do not function. They will sort themselves out after the fast.

On the second day of the fast you may feel more clear headed, but avoid the temptation to be more physically active, as you may have a sense of increased energy. Keep to the same resting mode and have the same liquid intake as on the previous day.

If you choose a 48-hour fast, then towards the end of the afternoon of the second day, despite the fact that you are not hungry, eat a baked or raw grated apple (eat very slowly and chew very well), or a small bowl of live, low-fat yogurt, or a bowl of thin homemade vegetable soup.

Several hours later have the same again or a little more of one of the other choices.

By the next morning you can resume normal eating, but you are bound to want smaller quantities.

If you do this over a weekend, starting on Friday evening and breaking the fast on Sunday afternoon, your working week will not be disturbed.

If you have opted for a 72-hour fast, then simply stretch the guidelines above into a third day and break the fast in precisely the same manner.

This sort of fast is appropriate once every three weeks or so, with cleansing, detox days or weekends in between indicated by your health status.

As time goes by, the reactions to the fast will lessen, so that your tongue will not get furred and your breath will stay sweet, and the odd symptoms will minimize of vanish.

As this happens, general health and well-being should be noticeably better.

If you wish to conduct a longer fast than that described above you must get professional advice on its suitability for you and on the protocols involved.

LONG FAST

(NOT RECOMMENDED UNLESS SUPERVISED)

Long fasting has an excellent record, for example:

- 'Dramatic' relief of patients poisoned by toxic cooking oil in Japan after between seven and 10 days of fasting (*American Journal of Industrial Medicine*, 5:147–153, 1984).

- Acute pancreatitis was helped more by fasting than by regular medication or any other form of treatment (*Digestion*, 30:224–230, 1984).

- Chances of recovery from auto-immune diseases such as

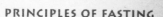

glomerulonephritis were enhanced by fasting (*Lancet* i:760–763, 1958), as were the conditions of patients with rheumatoid arthritis (*Clinical Ecology*, 2:3; 137–144, 1984).

In essence a long fast is simply an extended short fast. For this to be applied safely there needs to be a careful taking of a case history, a physical examination, evaluation and assessment of the chief complaint(s), followed by a decision as to whether or not fasting is the way forward. A fully compliant and willing patient is an absolute necessity, as is the need for full supervision.

For this a pleasant and safe environment is needed, as the home is not suitable for all the reasons of safety mentioned previously. Keeping a daily record of progress and vital signs is essential.

An adequate supply of suitable water is necessary, and attendants should be available at all times. Care over the progression and termination of the fast needs to be exercised.

In Switzerland, Scandinavia, Germany and Austria in particular, there are numerous spas and clinics which specialize in fasting. In the UK and the USA there are some similar establishments. However, the tendency has been away from water-only fasting towards juice-fasting in these countries, not for reasons of efficacy but mainly because of the cost of provision of supervision and monitoring.

Long fasts (water-only or modified) should never be undertaken at home unless supervision is assured by a suitably qualified health care professional.

THE ARGONNE FOUR-DAY ANTI-JET-LAG DIET/FAST

Dr Charles Ehret of Argonne National Laboratory, Division of Biological and Medical Research[20] has developed a pattern of feasting/fasting which regulates the traveller's internal clock to minimize the effects of jet-lag, and increasingly to speed up the adjustment time of shift-workers who periodically are required to rotate their working hours.

In discussing what a 'fast' means in the context of this diet we are told: 'Fast days help to deplete the liver's store of carbohydrates and prepare the body's clock for resetting.'

Coffee (and cola, tea and other caffeinated drinks) – Rules: On both feast days and the first fast day (days 1, 2 and 3 of the diet) coffee is allowed only between 3 and 5 pm, while on the second fast day (day 4 of the diet) coffee should be consumed if desired only in the morning when travelling west and between 6 and 11 pm when travelling east.

(Author's note: You would be much better without caffeine at all.)

On 'fast days' (days 1 and 4) you are instructed to eat light meals such as salads, light soups, fruits and juices.

Feast days (days 1 and 3 of the 4-day diet) involve a hearty high-protein breakfast and lunch, plus a high carbohydrate supper.

The recommended steps are as follows:

1) Make sure of the breakfast time at your destination and use this as a guide as to when to start the four-day diet, which should begin four days before the day of arrival at your destination.

2) On days one and three, eat a hearty breakfast and lunch (high protein – with eggs, meat, fish, high protein cereals and green beans recommended choices).

On these days, eat a carbohydrate evening meal (pasta or pancakes, potatoes or other starchy vegetables – but no meat) and a

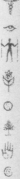

sweet desert (melon, grapes, etc.). Observe the coffee rules as described above.

3) On day two, eat a light salad, fruit, thin soup snacks only – and observe the same coffee rules.

4) On the fourth day, another fast day, take care of the revised coffee rules as described for this day.

If at all possible sleep on the flight until the normal breakfast time of your destination country, but no later. Have no alcohol on the flight.

Break the fast with a high protein breakfast – at what would be breakfast time at your destination, no matter what 'real' time this is for you, and continue thereafter to eat the day's meals according to the mealtimes at your destination.

Stay active and awake after breakfast and you should be synchronized with the local time and suffer no negative jet-lag effects.

In the next chapter I evaluate some of the associated methods which can assist the effectiveness of fasting, and which can make the process more comfortable.

ASSISTING DETOXIFICATION

For a fast or detoxification diet to be effective it is important that you are comfortable during the process. It also makes sense to try to enhance the efficiency and efficacy of the fast by encouraging other, normal, routes of detoxification – such as the skin, the bowels and the lungs – to work more efficiently at the same time.

In Chapter 5 descriptions were given of Dr Loomis's liver flush method as an essential part of his detoxification programme, and of Tom Moule's suggested use of various salts as a start to a detoxification diet, and these should be referred to alongside the outlines in this chapter for enhanced detoxification and improved liver function.

The summary of methods in this chapter are not comprehensive, but those described are of proven value, and impose little additional stress or effort in their application.

HOW OFTEN?

The various suggested methods will be presented in order of the ideal frequency of application rather than in any order of importance, which could well vary from individual to individual. For example, relaxation and stretching exercises are suggested daily, and if possible twice daily – for around 15 to 20 minutes at a time, while the use of an Epsom salts bath is suggested once weekly at most, as it can be somewhat enervating. This does not mean that relaxation is more or less important than the bath, simply that for practical reasons one is ideal if used regularly and the other infrequently.

BREATHING AND RELAXATION EXERCISES

These should be performed daily during a fast and the pre and post fast days, and if possible twice daily on all days. Breathing exercises should precede and continue onto a relaxation exercise so that they form a continuous sequence.

The purpose of the breathing exercise is:

- To encourage deeper and more rhythmic breathing which enhances lymphatic flow (the lymphatic system is a major element in the waste disposal system in the body).

- To provide a useful liver massage, from deep diaphragmatic movement during the exercise.

- To encourage greater elimination via the lungs (a good deal of toxic waste is eliminated via the lungs as we exhale).

- To improve oxygenation of tissues – important during the regeneration and repair processes which detoxification and fasting encourage.

- To allow for more effective relaxation following the practice of rhythmic breathing as described below.

The purpose of the relaxation exercise is:

- To encourage the energy saving which more relaxed muscles offer.

- To enhance immune function – something which is a major by-product of relaxation.

- To allow the mind to be more calm – something which is very important during the 'physiological rest' period offered by fasting and detoxification.

BREATHING SUGGESTIONS

There are many exercises to help improve breathing but there is just one which has been shown in medical studies to effectively reduce anxiety levels. This is an exercise based on traditional yogic pranayama breathing. The pattern is as follows:

1) Having placed yourself in a comfortable (ideally seated) position with your hands resting on your abdomen, just above your navel and just below your lower ribs, you inhale fully while counting to yourself up to no more than three (ideally two).

Translated into practical terms this means that you fill your lungs fairly quickly. The counting is necessary because the timing of the inhalation and exhalation phase of breathing is important in this exercise.

The inhalation should be accompanied by a sense that your abdomen is pushing your hands slightly forwards (as the diaphragm descends).

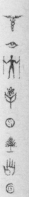

2) Without pausing to hold the breath at all, you then exhale fully taking four, five or even six seconds to do so (again you count to yourself at the same speed as when you inhaled).

As you breathe out you should have a sense of your hands coming back to where they started, as the abdominal protrusion deflates.

3) Repeat the inhalation (two seconds) and the exhalation (taking at least twice as long to exhale as you took to inhale). All inhalation should be through the nose if possible, while exhalation can be through nose or mouth. It is most important that the breathing out must be slow and continuous. It is no use breathing the air out in two seconds and then simply waiting until the count reaches five or six before inhaling again.

4) Repeat the cycles of inhalation/exhalation no less than 20 times, which should take no more than three to four minutes. By the time you have completed these 20 cycles you should feel calm and relaxed.

MODIFIED AUTOGENIC RELAXATION METHOD

Autogenic Training – a system of deep relaxation – is best learned from a fully trained instructor. However, the following modified form is an excellent way of achieving the objectives listed above.

Ideally this should follow on from the breathing exercise described above.

1) Lie on the floor or bed in a comfortable position (with perhaps a small cushion under your head), your eyes closed and knees bent if that makes your back feel easier.

2) Focus attention on your right arm or hand and silently say to yourself 'my right arm (or hand) feels heavy'. Try to *see* the arm relaxed and heavy, its weight sinking into the surface it is resting on. *Feel* its weight.

Over a period of about a minute, repeat the 'heavy arm' affirmation several times and try to stay focused on the weight and heaviness of your arm.

You are bound to lose focus as your attention wanders from time to time. A major part of the 'training' in the exercise is to stay focused, so don't feel angry – just go back to the arm and its heaviness. You may or may not be able to sense the heaviness, and this doesn't matter too much at first. If you do sense it, stay with it and enjoy the sense of release and letting go that comes with it.

3) Next, focus on your left arm or hand and do exactly the same thing for about a minute.

4) Move to your left leg and then your right leg, with similar timing, affirmations and focused attention.

5) Go back to your right arm or hand, and affirm that you sense a greater degree of warmth in that limb – 'my arm (or hand) is feeling warm (or hot)'.

6) After a minute or so, go to your left arm or hand, then your left leg and finally your right leg, each time with the

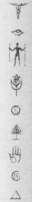

warming message and focused attention. If you sense warmth, stay with it for a while and feel it spread. Enjoy it.

7) Finally, focus on your forehead and affirm that it feels cool and refreshed. Stay with this refreshing sensation for a minute before completing the exercise with a clenching and unclenching of your fists, and a stretching of your arms. This breaks the self-induced state of deep relaxation and brings you back to present time. By repeating the whole exercise at least once a day during a fast, and on the days before and after it (10 to 15 minutes is all it will take) you will gradually find you can stay focused on each region and sensation (warmth, heaviness, coolness) for the full minute in each case, with profound benefits in terms of relaxation, energy conservation and immune function enhancement.

SKIN FRICTION

There are two good ways to encourage more effective elimination of toxic wastes through the skin, both suitable for use during a fast.

- Skin brushing: Daily frictioning of the skin before bathing or showering enhances skin function and the elimination process.

- The salt glow: A skin friction, using wet coarse (sea) salt or Epsom salts, before a bath or shower is particularly beneficial for people who have difficulty sweating or who have poor circulation to their hands and/or feet. It is also useful for people prone to rheumatic aches and pains. Skin brushing is probably less 'messy' and less arduous in its application than the salt glow method, but the latter is probably more efficient in encouraging the skin's elimination process. However, don't use this method more than once a week.

SKIN BRUSHING

It's a good idea to get into the habit of performing this 3 to 4 minute routine every day (except on days you are having an Epsom salts bath or are using the salt glow method – see below) while your skin is dry before washing yourself in a shower or bath. It helps you to shed the outer 'dead' layer of skin, encourages local circulation and improves your skin's potential to eliminate toxic waste.

Using a bath-mit, skin-brush or loofah (obtainable from any pharmacist) for your legs and arms, and a rough towel for your back, rub the main areas firmly enough to produce a red reaction but not hard enough to irritate your skin.

Sitting on a stool or the edge of the bath and starting slowly, gently perform a series of circular motions which do not overlap so that you slowly 'creep' the frictional rubbing up a leg or arm, taking special care not to brush anywhere that a skin rash exists or to put too much pressure onto tender skin areas such as your inner thigh, neck or breast.

Pay particular attention to your legs and arms with a brush/mit/loofah and your back and trunk with a towel. Although a towel produces a lesser reaction, it is more convenient for inaccessible areas such as your back.

This is something you should continue doing as a regular part of your bathing pattern between detox/fast days.

THE SALT GLOW METHOD

This is particularly useful for people who have difficulty in sweating, and it can be used instead of the Epsom salts bath

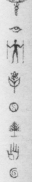

(see below). Near the start (within the first few days) of any detoxification programme and no more than once a week, instead of the daily skin brushing, use a salt-glow to produce a marked increase in the circulation to the skin, as well as a means of removing skin 'debris' and encouraging elimination and sweating.

Caution: Diabetics who use insulin, and people with cardio-vascular disease or who have open skin lesions should not use the salt glow method.

Sit on a stool which has been placed inside the shower or bath and place a cupful of salt (coarse is better, sea salt is best, but table salt will do). Moisten the salt with just enough water to make the grains stick together. Using about a tablespoon of salt at a time in each hand, rub this onto the skin of one leg, starting near your foot and working upwards. Use more salt as you need it and gradually treat one leg, then the other, and the same with your arms.

Next, friction as much of your back as you can easily reach (or have your partner or a friend do this for you), and finally your abdomen and chest. Avoid breast tissue.

After the salt friction, rinse with warm (not hot) water, ideally using a hand-held shower head. Rub your skin with your hands to rinse the salt off completely, and then briskly rub dry. It is suggested you then go straight to bed and keep yourself well-covered.

Perspiration may begin and become profuse, although as your detoxification programme progresses this will be less obvious. You should sleep very deeply. It is suggested that, for optimum skin health, you continue to use a salt glow once a week or fortnight, between detox or fasting periods.

Near the start (within the first few days) of any detoxification programme, and no more than once a week, instead of skin brushing or a salt glow, you might have an Epsom salts bath. The effects are similar to those expected from a salt glow – perspiration and enhanced detoxification through the skin – but they are more powerful. The same cautions as listed in the instructions for a salt glow should, therefore, be heeded, and the method should not be used by anyone who is frail or weak.

Place between 0.5 lb and 1 lb (225g–450g) of commercial Epsom salts (magnesium sulphate – available from most pharmacies), as well as 0.25 lb (112g) of sea salt, into a hot bath.

Soak in this for not less than 10 and not more than 20 minutes, topping up the hot water from time to time. Do not try to wash, as no lather can form because of the salts (similar to those found in the Dead Sea). Get out, dry yourself briskly and go to bed.

As with a salt glow, you will probably sweat and sleep heavily. Have drinking water readily available, as you may feel very thirsty. Apply a moisturizer to your skin next morning to avoid undue dryness, and clean the bath thoroughly to ensure the salt is removed.

NEUTRAL BATH

A neutral bath is one in which the water temperature is the same as your body temperature. It has a relaxing influence on the nervous system, and it is often used in cases of anxiety, stress, chronic pain and insomnia. By means of hydrostatic pressure it is also ideal for reducing excessive fluid retention.

Contraindications: In cases of skin conditions which react badly to water, or where there is serious cardiac disease.

A bath thermometer (obtainable from any pharmacy) is a necessary piece of equipment.

Run a full bath, with the water as close to 97°F (36.1°C) as possible, and certainly *not* exceeding that.

Immersion in water at this neutral temperature has a profoundly relaxing, sedating effect and a calming influence on nervous system activity. Get into the bath so that, if possible, water covers your shoulders, and support your head on a towel or sponge. The thermometer should be in the bath and the temperature should not be allowed to drop below 92°F (33.3°C). It can be topped up periodically but must not exceed the 97°F (36.1°C) limit. The duration of the bath can be anything from 30 minutes to several hours – the longer the better as far as the relaxation effects are concerned.

After the bath, pat dry quickly and get into bed for at least an hour. You can have a neutral bath whenever you feel anxious, restless or in need of a means to prepare yourself for sleep.

AROMATHERAPY

The selection of oils described below have proven herbal properties – *none is meant to be consumed*. Anyone who is pregnant should take professional advice before using aromatherapy oils.

When being added to a bath the oils are used neat in the running water which disperses and mixes them. If used for massage they should be combined with a neutral carrier oil.

Basil

On its own it can be used (20 drops in a bath) to treat weakness, fatigue (including mental tiredness/fogginess), headaches, nausea, feelings of tension or faintness and depression.

Chamomile

It can be used on its own (20 drops in a bath) to treat sleep and digestive disturbances, skin conditions, neuralgia and

inflammation. Combined with sage for menopausal problems
(10 drops of each in a bath).

Cypress

It can be used alone (20 drops in a bath) to treat rheumatic and muscular conditions, coughs, flu and nervous tension. Combined with Lavender – 20 drops of each in warm water for menopausal problems or for general nervous system treatment

Lavender

With cypress (as above) for menopausal or 'nervous system' problems, and with vetiver for anxiety (10 drops of each).

Neroli

Used alone (20 drops in a bath) to treat depression, insomnia, nervous tension and digestive upsets. Use together with basil (10 drops of each) in a bath in cases of anxiety, tension or depression.

ANTI-NAUSEA ACUPRESSURE POINT

The anti-nausea point is an acupressure point (known as Pericardium 6 in Traditional Chinese Medicine) which lies on the front of the wrist. It has been found – in medical studies conducted by Professor Dundee at Queen's University, Belfast – to markedly reduce nausea, no matter what the cause. It has been successfully used in treating the nausea of pregnancy (morning sickness); nausea which accompanies the use of chemotherapy and anaesthetics, and also travel sickness nausea).

The point is found on the centre of the palm side of the wrist, the width of two thumbs (your thumb) towards the elbow from the main crease of the wrist, between the two main tendons which run up your forearm. Press firmly onto the point (it will be tender) with your other thumb for up to a minute at a time whenever you have a sense of nausea – as is common in the early stages of detoxification.

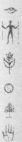

Note: Reread the details of Dr Loomis's liver flush, described in Chapter 5, as this is an additional method for reducing nausea by helping the liver to reduce its toxic load. Another alternative is the coffee enema which is described below.

THE USE OF ENEMAS

I have mentioned before that some of the leading experts in the use of fasting recommend enemas before and during both regular fasting and detoxification, while other experts insist that on a water-only fast it is unnecessary.

Based on my own experience over the past 35 years of practice as a naturopath, my recommendation is that if on any of the detoxification diets or modified fasts, constipation occurs – i.e. there is no bowel movement for more than two days – then a self-applied water enema or a colonic irrigation performed by an expert should be applied.

On a water-only fast I suggest that no enemas be used unless there is a history of bowel stasis (chronic constipation) in which case a self-applied water enema, or a colonic irrigation performed by an expert, should be considered before the start of the fast.

Anyone considering a long water-only or juice/broth fast will by now have understood that these should only be undertaken under supervision. Whoever is offering that supervision should advise you on their thoughts regarding the use of enemas, colonic irrigation, etc., and you can then make up your own mind, after consideration of the advice Method for water enema.

Caution: Anyone with a tendency to bleeding from the rectum should not use an enema (water or coffee). A health expert should be consulted before an enema is given to a child or to anyone who is elderly, frail, very ill, has bowel disease, hypertension or who is pregnant.

Buy a fountain syringe from a pharmacy. Lying on your right side on a towel, and having lubricated the end of the applicator with a sterile jelly, slowly ease the end of the tube past the anus into the rectum. Slowly squeeze the syringe containing water (*at body heat*) and over a period of several minutes take about a quart (1 litre) of water into the lower bowel. Do not rush the intake as cramp is possible. If you sense discomfort, stop squeezing and gently massage the abdomen until this passes.

Turn onto your left side once you have taken in the water and rest for a few minutes.

After at least five minutes of retention void the water into the toilet.

An alternative method is to use a gravity bag. This, containing about a quart (1 litre) of warm water, should be hung about two feet above the surface on which you are lying. Insert the applicator as described above, while lying on your right side. Release the clamp which allows water to flow down the tube and let this flow into your rectum. If there is discomfort, clamp off the tube and massage the abdomen. Once all the water has been taken in, turn onto your left side for a few minutes.

After five minutes void the water into the toilet.

COFFEE ENEMA

The coffee enema is designed to stimulate the liver into eliminating toxic debris in the bile. Take three tablespoons of ground (not instant) coffee and a quart (1 litre) of water. Boil for three minutes and allow the liquid to stand for 15 minutes. Use a quarter of this (half a pint/285ml) at body heat as an enema (using one of the methods described above) as often as you feel the need to ease nausea.

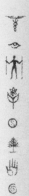

Lymphatic drainage massage, regular massage, shiatsu massage, osteopathic or chiropractic treatment – all are ideal optional accompaniments to a detoxification programme.

A regular massage is probably the most easily accessible, as many people have now acquired at least the basic skills for application of relaxation massage, although clearly a treatment from a qualified therapist/practitioner is preferable.

It is suggested that anyone undertaking a detox programme should get professional bodywork as often as it is available.

Stretching (yoga type) exercises are highly recommended and should be practised daily during any detoxification programme, as this enhances lymph flow, circulation and general well-being. There are many books and classes which can help in acquiring the basic skills for the use of stretching exercises.

THE SPIRITUAL DIMENSION

T he Bible tells us that both Moses and Jesus fasted for 40 days in the wilderness as part of their own spiritual struggles, and there are numerous similar examples in the holy texts of different cultures and religions. Clearly, something happens on a lengthy fast which allows for a greater spiritual awareness or heightened degree of consciousness. Indeed, fasting as a spiritual exercise has roots and traditions which pass into prehistory.

Today many religious orders, in all traditions, still contain elements of fasting or abstention from what may be regarded as normal eating patterns as part of their disciplines. Many of the strict rules which apply to different holy orders, as well as the dietary changes, such as those involved in the Lent period, can be seen as modified rather than true fasting. But the fact that there are similar traditions in most religions and spiritual practices supports the suggestion that a change takes place, and perhaps the beginnings of an inner revolution occurs, when we voluntarily abstain from something as basic as eating and drinking for a period of time.

Muhammad Salim Khan, a Muslim physician practising in the United Kingdom, puts these changes into words which are

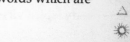

easily understood in his book *Islamic Medicine* (Routledge, Kegan and Paul, London, 1986):

> Complete fasting (sawm) is one institution that combines spiritual, physical, individual and community needs in a most harmonious way. The spiritual aspect of an individual is developed and enhanced in the most potent and sublime manner. Taqwa – God consciousness, discipline and empathy with the poor and needy – is the main emphasis behind fasting. Fasting is a devotional process and internal purification enables the person to transcend his gross physical needs.

He goes on to explain that the biological effects of fasting – detoxification and healing enhancement – are, of course, important and that the process involves a very personal commitment and effort, but it is clear that he (and Islam) consider the fasting process to be a means by which the individual achieves a closer link with his/her faith, spirituality, a higher consciousness, and therefore with his or her greater wellbeing.

Kahn stresses that despite the personal sacrifice involved, fasting is, in Islamic cultures, a community affair, since in the month of Ramadan almost the entire community take part in the rituals and events which accompany this special time. However, the young (prepubescent), the aged or extremely ill, as well as pregnant and lactating women, are advised to be cautious or to avoid the practice.

It is probably no coincidence that naturopathic thinking in general, and fasting in particular, are extremely widely used in Hindu societies, and that Yoga methodology which derives from that same ancient source involves variations on the theme of detoxification, since these methods grew out of traditional Ayurvedic medicine which takes a comprehensive mind/body/spirit view of the human condition.

Ayurveda aims at creation of a state of balance, and the means of achieving this often involves fasting. This process has an objective which leads towards an ideal in which we are not only able to 'cleanse, purify, and prevent disease, but also uplift oneself into a realm of awareness previously unknown,' states Vasant Lad, a practising physician at the Ayurvedic Institute of Albuquerque, New Mexico (quoted in *Alternative Medicine – The Definitive Guide*, Future Medicine Inc., San Francisco).

It may be thought that fasting for health is one thing, and fasting for spiritual reasons quite another. However, as Dr Kahn suggests, there is no reason at all why both benefits should not be available when we use this most ancient, basic and effective method of mind/body purification.

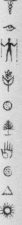

REFERENCES

CHAPTER 2

1   Arbesman, A. 'Fasting and Prophecy in Pagan and Christian Antiquity', *Tradition* 7:1–71, 1951.

2   Salloum, T. and Burton, A. 'Therapeutic fasting' in *Textbook of Natural Medicine* (Eds Pizzorno, J. and Murray, M.) Bastyr University, Seattle WA 1989.

3   Fuhrman, J. Fasting and Eating for Health, St Martin's Press, New York, 1995.

4   Report by Tom Paulson, *Seattle Post-Intelligencer*, Friday 30 June 1995.

5   'Dr Tanner's fast', *BMJ* 11:171, 1880.

6   Guelpa, G. 'Starvation and purgation in the relief of diabetes', *BMJ* ii:1050–1051.

7   Driscoll, C. and Loxterkamp, D. 'Fasting: The history, pathophysiology and complications', *Western Journal of Medicine*, 137:370–399, 1981.

8   Salloum, T. and Burton, A., op cit.

9   Allen, F. 'Prolonged fasting in diabetes', *American Journal of Medical Science*, 150:480–485.

10 Vessby, B. et al 'Improved metabolic control after supplemented fasting in overweight diabetic type 2 patients', *Acta Med Scand*, 216:67–74, 1984.

11 Lennox, W. and Cobb, S. 'Studies in Epilepsy', *Archives of Neurology and Psychiatry*, 20:711–779, 1928.

12 Stewart, W. et al 'Features of a successful therapeutic fast of 382 days duration', *Postgraduate Medical Journal* 49:203–209, 1973.

13 Goodhart, R. & Shils, M. *Modern Nutrition and Health and Disease*, Lea & Febiger, Philadelphia, 1980.

14 Gresham, G. *Atherosclerosis*, 23: 379–391, 1975.

15 Duncan, G. et al 'Contraindications and therapeutic results of fasting in obese patients', *Annals N.Y. Academy of Sciences* 131:632–636, 1965.

16 Navarro, S. et al 'Comparison of fasting, nasogastric suction and cimetidine in treatment of acute pancreatitis', *Digestion* 30:24–230, 1984.

17 Imamura, M. et al 'A trial of fasting cure for PCB poisoned patients in Taiwan', *American Journal of Industrial Medicine* 5:147–153, 1984.

18 Brod, J. et al 'Influence of fasting on the immunological reactions and course of acute glomerulonephritis', *Lancet* i: 760–763, 1958.

19 Kjeldsen-Kragh, J. et al 'Controlled trial of fasting and one year vegetarian diet in rheumatoid arthritis', *Lancet* 338:899–902, 1991.

20 Panush, R. 'Controversial arthritis remedies', *Bulletin of Rheumatic Diseases*, 34:1–10, 1985.

21 Fuhrman, J., op cit.

22 Shigemasa, C. et al 'Effect of vegetarian diet on SLE', *Lancet* 339:1177, 1992.

23 Wofy, D. 'New approaches to treating SLE', *Western Journal of Medicine*, 147:181–186, 1987.

24 Lithell, H. et al 'A fasting and vegetarian diet treatment of chronic inflammatory disorders', *Acta Dermato-Venerologia* (Stockholm), 63:397, 1983.

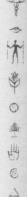

25 Riordan, A. et al 'Treatment of active Crohn's disease by exclusion diet', *Lancet* 342:1131–1134, 1993.

26 Lithell, H. et al, op cit.

27 Sizuki, J. et al 'Fasting therapy for psychosomatic disease', *Tohoku Journal of Experimental Medicine*, 118 (sup): 245–259, 1976.

28 Boehme, D. et al 'Preplanned fasting in the treatment of mental disease – Survey of current Soviet literature', *Schizophrenia Bulletin*, 3:2:288–296, 1977.

29 Cott, A. *Fasting: The ultimate diet*, Bantam Books, New York, 1975.

CHAPTER 3

1 Salloum, T. 'Fasting – Patient Guidelines', *Textbook of Natural Medicine* (eds Pizzorno, J. and Murray, M.) Bastyr University, Seattle, WA, 1987.

2 Weindruch, R. and Walford, R. *The Retardation of Aging by Dietary Restriction*, Charles Thomas, Springfield, Illinois, 1988.

3 Chaitow, L. *Natural Life Extension*, Thorsons, London, 1992.

4 Burton, A. 'Fasting too long', *Health Science*, 2:144–146, 1979.

5 Cubberley, P. et al 'Lactic acidosis and death after treatment of obesity by fasting', *New England Journal of Medicine*, 272:628–630, 1965.

6 Norbury, F. 'Contraindications to long-term fasting', *JAMA*, 1964.

7 Kahan, A. 'Death after therapeutic starvation', *Lancet* i:1378–1379, 1968.

8 Salloum, T. and Burton, A. 'Therapeutic fasting', *Textbook of Natural Medicine*, (eds Pizzorno, J. and Murray, M.) Bastyr University, Seattle. WA, 1987.

9 Stewart, W. 'Fragmentation of cardiac myofibrils after therapeutic starvation', *Lancet* i:1154, 1969.

10 Fuhrman, J. MD *Fasting and Eating for Health*, St Martin's Press, NY, 1995.

CHAPTER 4

1 Salloum, T. and Burton, A. 'Therapeutic fasting' *Textbook of Natural Medicine*, (eds Pizzorno, J. and Murray, M.) Bastyr University, Seattle, WA, 1987.

2 Elkeles, R. and Tavill, A. *Biochemical Aspects of Human Disease*, Blackwell, Boston, MA, 1983.

3 White, A. et al *Principles of Biochemistry* (6th edition), McGraw-Hill, New York, 1978.

4 Owen, O. et al 'Brain metabolism during fasting' *Journal of Clinical Investigation*, 46:1589–1595, 1967.

5 Fasting section in *Alternative Medicine – The Definitive Guide*, Future Medicine Publishing, Puyallup, WA, 1994.

6 Airola, P. *Health Secrets from Europe*, Arco Publishing, New York, 1975.

7 Balch, J. and P. *Prescription for Nutritional Healing*, Avery Publishing, Garden City Park, NY 1990.

8 Fuhrman, J. *Fasting and Eating for Health*, St Martin's Press, New York, 1995.

9 Chaitow, B. Personal correspondence.

CHAPTER 5

1 Davies, S. and Stewart, A. *Nutritional Medicine*, Pan, London, 1987.

2 Chaitow, L. *Clear Body Clear Mind*, Gaia, London, 1989.

3 Lake, S. and Mayne, S. *The 10-day Brown Rice Diet*, Wellspring, London, 1990.

4 Chaitow, B. *My Healing Secrets*, Health Science Press, 1980

5 Moule, T. *Handbook of Nature Cure*, Champneys Resort, Tring, 1962.

6 Barrie, S. 'Food Allergy Testing', in *Textbook of Natural*

Medicine (eds Pizzorno and Murray) Bastyr University Seattle, 1989

7   Chaitow, L. *Stone Age Diet*, Macdonald Optima, London, 1989.

8   Airola, P. *Health Secrets from Europe*, Arco Publishing, New York, 1975.

9   Salloum, T. and Burton, A. 'Therapeutic Fasting', in *Textbook of Natural Medicine* (eds Pizzorno and Murray), Bastyr University, Seattle, 1989.

10 Rauch, E. *Naturopathic Treatment of Colds and Infectious Diseases*, Haug, Brussels, 1991.

11 Lust, John B. *Raw Juice Therapy*, Thorsons, Wellingborough, 1976.

12 In 'Fasting', *Alternative Medicine – The Definitive Guide*, (Med. ed. L. Chaitow), Future Medicine Publications, Puyallup, WA, 1994.

13 Gerson, S. *Ayurveda*, Element Books, Shaftsbury, Dorset, 1993.

14 Mayr, F. X. *Fundamentals of the diagnosis of digestive illnesses*, Goisern (Ober-Oisterreich) Verlag Neues Leben, 1921.

15 Rauch, E. *Intestinal Cleansing According to F. X. Mayr*, Haug, Heidelberg, 1982.

16 Newman Turner, R. *Naturopathic Medicine*, Thorsons, Wellingborough, 1984.

17 In 'Fasting' *Alternative Medicine – The Definitive Guide*, (Med. ed. L. Chaitow), Future Medicine Publications, Puyallup, WA, 1994.

18 Waerland, A. and E. *Health is Your Birthright*, Humata Publishing, Switzerland.

19 Moyle, A. 'The Guelpa fast', *British Naturopathic Journal*, Volume 7, Number 10, 1969.

20 Argonne National Laboratory, 9700 South Cass Avenue, Argonne, Illinois 60439 – as reported in Holiday Inn Handbook, Countryside-La-Grange, 1995.

RESOURCES

NATUROPATHS

Naturopaths are the practitioners most likely to have trained in the use of therapeutic fasting. Contact one of the organizations listed below for information about their membership lists as well as for the addresses of clinics which may offer naturopathic care and advice.

The British Naturopathic Association (General Council and Register of Naturopaths) represents the majority of qualified UK naturopaths.

The British Natural Hygiene Society represents trained individuals whose expertise in fasting is probably the highest in Europe. However, there are relatively few of these.

Most members of the College of Osteopaths Practitioners Association are also qualified naturopaths, and many Nutrition Counsellors are also familiar with fasting methods.

It is suggested that you enquire directly about the training of whoever you contact and ask specifically about their fasting expertise before consulting them.

Fasting, detoxification and elimination diets are widely prescribed and utilised, usually under expert supervision, at health hydros in the UK and Europe. Individual enquiries should be made as to the costs involved and to ascertain whether what is on offer is appropriate to your particular needs.

British Naturopathic Association
6 Netherhall Gardens
London NW3 5RR
(Phone: 0171–435–6464)

Incorporated Society of Registered Naturopaths
1 Albamarle Road
The Mount
York YO2 1EN

College of Osteopaths Practitioners Association
13 Furzehill Road
Borehamwood
Herts WD6 2DG
(Phone: 0181–905–1937)

British Natural Hygiene Society
Shalimar
First Avenue
Frinton-on-Sea
Essex CO13 9EZ
(Phone: 01255–672823)

Council for Nutrition Education and Therapy
34 Wadham Road
London SW15 2LR

Society for the Promotion of Nutritional Therapy
PO Box 47
Heathfield
East Sussex TN21 8ZX
(Phone: 01435–867007)

Register of Nutritional Therapists
Hatton Green
Warwick CV35 7LA
(Phone: 01926–484449)

For information about a Colonic Hydrotherapist contact:
Colonic International Association
16 New England Lane
London NW3 4TG
(Phone: 0171–483–1595)

For books and products (essential oils, herbs, nutritional supplies etc.) which you may need during detoxification, contact
your local health food store or The Nutri Centre, 7 Park
Crescent, London W1N 3HE (Phone: 0171–436–5122) who offer
a next-day mail order service.

INDEX

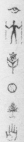